THE FORMULA

BY GENE AND JOYCE DAOUST

40-30-30 Fat Burning Nutrition

The Formula

THE
FORMULA

A PERSONALIZED 40-30-30
WEIGHT LOSS PROGRAM

Since 1990 it has been our mission to change the way Americans view nutrition. We also want to help as many people as possible in their quest to burn fat and lose weight. We hope you find this book useful in helping you achieve all of your goals.

KEEP THE FAITH AND THINK BIG.

GENE AND JOYCE DAOUST

BALLANTINE BOOKS   NEW YORK

A Ballantine Book
Published by The Ballantine Publishing Group
Copyright © 2001 by Gene Daoust and Joyce Daoust

All rights reserved under International and Pan-American Copyright Conventions. Published in the United States by The Ballantine Publishing Group, a division of Random House, Inc., New York, and simultaneously in Canada by Random House of Canada Limited, Toronto.

Ballantine and colophon are registered trademarks of Random House, Inc.

www.randomhouse.com/BB/

Library of Congress Catalog Card Number: 00-110516

ISBN 0-345-44305-5

Manufactured in the United States of America

First Edition: January 2001

10 9 8 7 6 5 4 3 2 1

THIS BOOK IS DEDICATED TO GENE'S PARENTS.

"I MISS YOU MORE THAN EVER."

CONTENTS

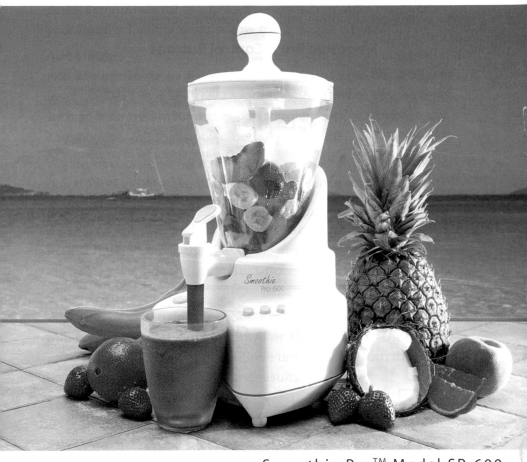

Smoothie Pro™ Model SP-600

Back to Basics Products, Inc.
11660 South State Street
Draper, Utah 84020
801-571-7349 • fax 801-571-6061
www.backtobasicsproducts.com

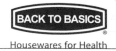

BACK TO BASICS

Housewares for Health

Instructions

Smoothie
Pro 600™

BACK TO BASICS®

PART FOUR: TROUBLESHOOTING

PART FIVE: MOTIVATIONAL TOOLS

ACKNOWLEDGMENTS

What a long strange trip it's been.
—The Grateful Dead

It has been a very strange trip indeed. We are very proud of the work we have done to make the 40-30-30 Formula popular, and we are glad it has helped millions of people. Along the way, some key individuals have helped us.

First, we would like to thank Don and Marjorie Tyson, two of the world's experts in amino acids. Their early training in protein and amino acids helped us to accept the unaccepted and was the foundation that helped us start the 40-30-30 revolution.

A very special thanks to Dr. Barry Sears, who in our opinion is one of the world's greatest minds in nutrition. With his training in the science of essential fatty acids and dietary endocrinology, he has helped us more than anyone else, and there are millions of people whose lives are better because of his work. We would also like to thank Doug Sears for his business help in the early days at our clinic, the BioSyn Human Performance Center. A special thanks to Meg, Steve, Jennifer, Candy, and all of our staff for their hard work there.

ACKNOWLEDGMENTS

Because there are too many to list individually, we want to thank all of the doctors, pharmacists, trainers, nutritionists, athletes, and other health professionals from the Pacific Northwest with whom we worked over the past fifteen years. Their input has been invaluable and it continues to help us. Also, a special thanks to personal trainers Donald Baker and Pete Seaman. They were two of the first strength professionals to grasp the 40-30-30 concept, and their continued dedication as well as their incredible natural physiques are an inspiration to us all. We also want to thank Seattle pharmacist George Stimac and his son John, who were dedicated pioneers.

We want to thank Balance Bar company founders Tom Davidson and Dick Lamb and company president Jim Wolf, as well as all of the other Balance staff we worked with. Your dedication in marketing a quality nutrition bar helped us to develop a better 40-30-30 program. Thanks to all of the early Balance team, especially Michael Sanchez and Phil and Donna Leclair, who stuck in there through the tough times. We want to thank Sheri Sears, Bill Logue, and all of the staff at PR Nutrition and *Ironman*, who had an uphill battle to convert endurance athletes and made it to the top.

In addition, our thanks go to New Vision International and all of their team members for all their support.

We thank all of those who responded to our first book, *40-30-30 Fat Burning Nutrition*. Your kind words, comments, and success stories continue to inspire and motivate us as well as help us to develop better programs.

We thank our agents, David Vigliano and Dean Williamson, as well as our editor, Maureen O'Neal, and everyone at Ballantine Books. Your confidence has helped us write a truly awesome book that can help millions!

WHO ARE
JOYCE AND GENE DAOUST?

Married since 1985, Joyce and Gene Daoust are the clinical nutritionists who worked with Dr. Barry Sears in developing and testing the original 40-30-30 zone nutrition program. In the early 1990s, the Daousts owned and operated the BioSyn Human Performance Center, a cutting-edge weight loss and sports nutrition center located in Kirkland, Washington, and the world's first 40-30-30 zone nutrition clinic. It was there the 40-30-30 zone nutrition craze began to take off. The Daousts were also the key nutritionists who helped develop the programs for the leading 40-30-30 Nutrition Bar manufacturers.

Joyce and Gene are two of America's leading experts in nutrition, fitness, and weight loss. They are both dynamic and highly sought-after motivational speakers and nutrition trainers. They have a wonderful ability to make the 40-30-30 fat burning system easy to understand and implement, as well as to inspire all types of individuals to take action that will quickly and easily help them to look, feel, and perform better. They are authors of the book *40-30-30 Fat Burning Nutrition*, which has sold approximately 400,000 copies.

Joyce and Gene have been featured on more than five hundred television and radio shows and in magazines, newspapers, and other publications. The Daousts conduct programs for athletic teams and groups, professional trade associations, corporations and sales organizations, physicians, and health professionals.

The Daousts have traveled the country lecturing on 40-30-30 nutrition. Since 1990 the Daousts have helped more than 500,000 people use the 40-30-30 zone nutrition program to lose weight and feel and perform better, and their ultimate goal is to help millions.

WHY ANOTHER DIET BOOK?

In 1996, we wrote our first book, *40-30-30 Fat Burning Nutrition*, which for many made the 40-30-30 zone diet concept instantly comprehensible. Five years later we still get calls from doctors who want to know where they can find that book because it's the best way to explain 40-30-30 zone nutrition to their patients. Those same five years resulted in thousands of calls and letters. Clients have provided us with valuable information, success stories, and their favorite recipes, which we will share with you in *The Formula*.

The Formula takes *40-30-30 Fat Burning Nutrition* to the next level. We've learned that dieters love plain language and want plenty of great recipes to choose from, including family style meals and kids' favorites, all of which you'll now find in *The Formula*. *The Formula* expands on what readers loved about our first book without losing any of its simplicity.

The Formula features our 21-Day Fat Flush Formula. We originally developed the 40-30-30 Fat Flush Plan for bodybuilders and other athletes who were in their final six-week phase of "cutting up" before their competition. It was so successful that we began using it with all of our clients. Fat loss on the 21-Day Fat Flush Formula is so dramatic that dieters often ask if they can stay on it indefinitely. The answer to that is yes. The Fat Flush Formula is actually the best lifetime choice for a diabetic or a person who is hypoglycemic (with the advice of his or her physician). However, after using the Fat Flush Formula for the first 21 days, most people can combine Fat Flush meals with Regular Formula meals for continued weight loss or maintenance. We refer to that as your Formula for Life.

Fat Flush Formula meals contain the 40-30-30 ratio of 40% of calories from carbohydrates, 30% from protein, and 30% from fat. They differ from our Regular Formula meals in that the 40% carbohydrates they contain are from medium- to low-glycemic carbohydrates, whereas Regular meals offer a greater variety of both low- and high-glycemic carbohydrates. Fat Flush Formula meals provide adequate carbohydrates for brain function, prevent the possibility of ketosis, and severely tighten the control of blood sugar levels. This formula is ideal for those giving up their high-protein diets or for dieters who want to jump-start *The Formula* and maximize fat burning.

The Fat Flush Formula is a complete, personalized, simple plan that balances body chemistry to its highest fat burning potential. Each meal and snack contains the 40-30-30 fat burning ratio. So while you're eating generous meals, you never feel sluggish or hungry afterward. Depending on the amount of weight you have to lose, you can stay on the Fat Flush Formula until all of your excess weight disappears, or just jump-start your first 21 days.

Unlike all other one-size-fits-all diet books, *The Formula* is different in that it provides a personalized nutrition program and offers five different personalized meal planners, one just right for your specific gender, weight, and activity level. The A, B, and C plans are typically used by women, the C, D, and E plans by men. The Meal Plan Selection Chart on page 63 will help you determine which plan is right for you based on your beginning weight. As the pounds burn off, you may need to adjust your meal quantities by using a different meal plan. A well-balanced eating plan should be shared by your entire family. Simply determine which A, B, C, D, or E plan is right for each member of your family. Each plan provides appropriate portions and is simple to follow. You will also enjoy the convenience of our Family Style Meals as well as the Kids' Favorites.

If you think dessert is off-limits, think again. Included in *The Formula* are Joyce's famous Fat Burning Cheesecakes plus many other Fat Flush and Regular 40-30-30 dessert recipes. We'll show you how you can even choose to eat cheesecake for breakfast and snacks and still lose weight.

The Formula can work for everyone, even those who don't like to exercise, although those who do work out get even better results. We both love to exercise and highly recommend it as part of *The Formula*. We've even included our fresh new approach to exercise, the 40-30-30 Exercise Formula.

We've had people call to tell us they've tried every diet out there, and this is the first time they have ever seen such dramatic results while eating delicious meals and feeling great. Several women told us we should call the diet the Fat Melting Diet or the Miracle Diet or the Magic Potion Diet. We decided to write a personalized diet book, reflecting our combined experience of more than thirty years in weight loss and high-performance nutrition, and simply call it *The Formula*.

Part One

THE SCIENCE
MADE EASY

Chapter One

UNDERSTANDING BASIC HUMAN NUTRITION

THE SIX CLASSES OF ESSENTIAL NUTRIENTS

Your body requires six essential nutrient classes for growth, mainte-nance, and repair of its tissues. Essential nutrients are those that the body cannot make and must obtain from an outside source. To provide a well-balanced diet, the foods you eat must contain all of the essential nutri-ents in the amounts appropriate for good health. The challenge is to eat a balanced diet that provides these nutrients without overeating. A closer look at the nutrients helps you understand their importance as part of a balanced diet. The six classes of es-sential nutrients are carbohydrates, protein, fats, vitamins, minerals, and water.

The Six Classes of Essential Nutrients

1. *Carbohydrates*
2. *Protein*
3. *Fats*
4. *Vitamins*
5. *Minerals*
6. *Water*

Carbohydrates, proteins, and fats are classified as macronutrients and must be consumed in large amounts throughout the day. These energy-producing nutrients break down to supply calories (the measure of energy in food). One gram of carbohydrate equals four calories, one gram of protein also equals four calories, and one gram of fat equals nine calories.

Vitamins and minerals are classified as micronutrients. These essential organic and inorganic nutrients are found in the foods you eat and are vital to life. They act as cofactors and are critical for proper body function. Many foods today lack vitamins and minerals, having been grown in depleted soils or overprocessed. For this reason, we recommend supplementing your diet with a well-balanced vitamin and mineral capsule. Think of it as nutritional insurance.

Water, of course, is indispensable for life. This essential nutrient flows through every cell in your body, bringing in nourishment and taking wastes away. However, most people don't drink enough water. If you don't get enough water daily, you may experience heartburn, stomach cramps, low back pain, headache, and fatigue. But if you drink adequate amounts of water, your body runs more smoothly, your circulation is improved, your digestion enhanced, and your complexion brightened.

How much water you drink depends on your size and activity level. Rather than the standard eight 8-ounce glasses per day, try this method: Divide your weight by two and drink that many ounces of water per day. Thus for a woman weighing 130 pounds (130 ÷ 2 = 65) the eight 8-ounce glasses of water per day is right on target. However, a 200-pound man needs approximately 100 ounces per day, or about eight 12-ounce glasses per day.

Burning fat is also a very dehydrating process. Toxins are stored in fat cells, and as excess body fat is being burned for energy, these stored toxins enter the bloodstream. Water becomes the vehicle for transporting toxins from your body. Because of this process, water becomes even more important when you are burning fat and losing weight.

Determine your water requirements and challenge yourself to drink that amount of water daily. You will be amazed at how good you feel when you simply drink adequate amounts of pure water.

Years of experience working with thousands of people taught us that most people don't know which foods are classified as carbohydrates, proteins, or fats. That makes it difficult when you attempt to eat 40% of calories from carbohydrates, 30% from protein, and 30% from fat. The following is a simple review of the three groups of macronutrients. It can help you understand the unique characteristics of each of these essential nutrients and why it is important to include all of them in every meal you eat.

Although most foods contain a mixture of carbohydrates, proteins, and fats, we classify foods according to their predominant nutrient.

CARBOHYDRATES

Carbohydrates are found in virtually all plant foods. Fruits, vegetables, grains, legumes (beans), and starchy foods such as potatoes, rice, pasta, and bread consist primarily of carbohydrates. Add to that list sugary foods such as ice cream, cookies, cakes, candies, and pies, plus chips, pretzels, popcorn, soda pop, and juice, and

Body Weight/ Water Requirement Calculator

1. Total body weight   ____
2. Divide by 2   ____
3. Daily ounces per day   ____

you can see that you are bombarded with carbohydrate foods. In fact, there are very few people suffering from carbohydrate deficiency, unless, of course, they are in ketosis—but we'll discuss that later.

The primary role of carbohydrates is to supply energy to the body, or more important, to provide energy to the brain. No matter what form of carbohydrate, simple or complex, all carbohydrates convert into the same thing—blood sugar, more properly termed glucose. So, whether you eat a candy bar or pure sugar, an apple or whole wheat pasta, they all break down into the same thing: glucose.

If you eat a meal that is primarily carbohydrate, such as a bowl of cereal, juice, and toast, the level of glucose in your body will rise. When large amounts of glucose enter the bloodstream at one time, your blood sugar level rises and insulin is released to lower it. Elevated insulin levels force your body to burn glucose for energy instead of stored body fat. Even worse, elevated insulin levels convert excess carbohydrates into fat.

Problems also occur when carbohydrates are avoided (for example, eggs and bacon without toast or juice for breakfast). High protein, high fat, low carbohydrate diets can promote a sluggish feeling because the brain requires large amounts of glucose to maintain proper mental function. If you don't eat enough carbohydrates, blood sugar levels drop too low and the brain suffers.

The best sources of carbohydrates are foods that are high in fiber, low in starch, and low in sugar (low glycemic). We use low to medium glycemic carbohydrates in the 21-Day Fat Flush Formula meals. These high fiber carbohydrates are nutrient dense, which means they are naturally low in calories and high in vitamins and minerals. They should be your primary source of carbohydrates and will produce the best and fastest results.

Best High Quality Carbohydrate Sources

Fruits: *Apples, oranges, grapefruit, strawberries, pears, peaches, and plums*

Vegetables: *Broccoli, asparagus, green beans, cauliflower, zucchini, and spinach*

Grains: *Barley, oatmeal, rye, brown and wild rice, and whole wheat pasta*

Legumes: *Black beans, white beans, garbanzo beans, kidney beans, and lentils*

WHAT ARE YOUR CARBOHYDRATE REQUIREMENTS?

In the Formula, we use the revolutionary 40-30-30 nutrition ratio. Forty percent of your calories should come from carbohydrates. To determine your carbohydrate requirements, you must know that you will need one-third more carbohydrates than protein. We know most people don't like to work on math problems when they are hungry, so we have done this for you in the Macronutrient Chart (page 65).

PROTEIN

Protein foods are primarily foods that come from an animal source. The quality of a protein food is determined by two factors: the amino acid balance it contains and its digestibility. A complete protein contains all of the essential amino acids in relatively the same amount as humans require.

High quality protein sources should also be easy to digest and low in fat, making some of the best protein sources eggs (less some yolks), lowfat dairy products, skinless chicken and turkey, fish, and lean cuts of red meat. Lowfat soy products may also be included.

As protein is digested, long peptide chains begin to break down into amino acids, enter the bloodstream, and are rearranged into more than 50,000 new body proteins. Just as the letters of the alphabet can be arranged to create thousands of different words, the 22 commonly known amino acids are precisely arranged in the bloodstream to build thousands of necessary body proteins that make up, build, and repair the human body on a continuous basis. These body proteins include hair, skin, nails, blood, hormones, digestive and regulatory enzymes, muscle tissue, brain neurotransmitters, your immune system, and much more. Remember that *only* amino acids rebuild these vital body proteins.

If you consume adequate amounts of quality protein at every meal, a continuous supply of amino acids is available to build and repair your body. Protein in a meal also stimulates the release of glucagon, a fat burning hormone that maintains stable blood glucose levels and releases stored fat so it can be burned for energy.

Many people have heard that beans and rice are a good source of protein for vegetarians. When two plant foods, each containing the amino acids that the other lacks, are eaten at the same meal, they can

Best High Quality Protein Sources

- *Cottage cheese (lowfat and nonfat)*
- *Chicken and turkey (skinless)*
- *Eggs and egg whites*
- *Fish*
- *Lean meats*
- *Lowfat tofu and tempeh (soy products)*
- *Whey protein powder (90% pure)*

make a complete protein. However, a high quality protein must be not only complete but also digestible. The fibers found in plant foods wrap around the protein chains, making it difficult to digest and utilize the amino acids they contain. Besides, beans are 75% carbohydrates, and rice is 90%. So we consider beans and rice carbohydrate foods and recommend adding additional easy-to-digest high quality protein with these foods.

A low protein diet can cause amino acid imbalance, muscle loss, and decreased metabolism, and prevents the release of glucagon necessary for burning body fat.

But too much protein can also cause problems. A high protein diet can set you up for the abnormal metabolic state known as ketosis. Sure, the first week may bring your weight down, but be aware that at best a pound or two of what you lose is fat and the rest can be lean muscle, water weight, and mineral loss. Once the dieter goes off the diet, the weight can zoom back up, quite often to a point higher than before.

WHAT ARE YOUR PROTEIN REQUIREMENTS?

The Formula uses the revolutionary 40-30-30 nutrition ratio. Thirty percent of your calories come from protein. Your gender, size, and activity level determine how much protein you require. You need between .5 and 1 gram of protein per pound of lean muscle weight per day. We know most people don't like to work on math problems when they are hungry, so we have done this for you in the Macronutrient Chart (page 65).

FAT

The last of the three macronutrients is fat, certainly the most confusing of all. In the past you were told that fat is bad and to avoid it. Now you hear that there are good fats and bad fats. The most important point to remember is that fat is an essential nutrient and that we need it every day from an outside source. I often hear people say they don't need to eat any fat, since they already have plenty of it. The truth is, you need fat to burn fat.

To maintain good health and to burn fat, your diet must contain adequate amounts of fat sources that supply essential fatty acids. Essential fatty acids play a critical role in energy production, balancing hormones, controlling hunger, and stabilizing blood sugar. It is important to remember that fat in a meal slows the digestion of the meal so that it trickles into the bloodstream, keeping blood glucose levels normal.

Best High Quality Fat Sources

- *Olives and olive oil*
- *Avocados*
- *Almonds, walnuts, macadamia nuts, and pecans*
- *All types of raw nuts and seeds*
- *Fish and fish oils*
- *Vegetable oils*

The right kind of fat provides omega 3 and 6 fatty acids. These "good" fats are unprocessed and occur naturally in foods. Good sources are raw nuts and seeds, olives and avocados, and vegetable oils such as safflower, canola, and olive. Although fish is primarily thought of as a protein source, it also provides valuable EPA (eicosapentaenoic acid) fatty acids. Coldwater fish such as salmon, tuna, sardines, and mackerel are some of your best sources of fat.

A healthy diet should contains 30% of

its total calories from fat, with 10% of the total calories from saturated fat, 10% from unsaturated fat, and 10% from monounsaturated fat. Animal proteins contain saturated fats, vegetables and vegetable oils contain unsaturated fats, and avocados, olives, olive oil, nuts, and seeds contain monounsaturated fats.

The fats to avoid are called *trans fats* and are found in hydrogenated vegetable oils.

WHAT ARE YOUR FAT REQUIREMENTS?

The Formula uses the revolutionary 40-30-30 nutrition ratio. Thirty percent of your calories come from fat. We know most people don't like to work on math problems when they are hungry, so we have done this for you in the Macronutrient Chart (page 65).

SUMMARY

The key thing to remember about nutrition is balance. Balanced nutrition is the magic bullet to good nutrition. It always has been and it always will be, and the Formula is simply balanced nutrition made easy. The Formula is a balanced nutrition program personalized for your specific requirements. Each meal and snack contains the 40-30-30 ratio of carbohydrates, protein, and fat to fuel your body correctly. Every time you eat, the carbohydrates in the meal provide glucose for your brain and prevent ketosis. The protein provides amino acids needed to build and repair body proteins and releases glucagon, your fat burning hormone. And fat supplies the fatty acids critical for blood sugar control, appetite suppression, and hormone production.

The Formula

40% Carbohydrates
- *To provide fuel for your brain*
- *To prevent ketosis*

30% Protein
- *To provide amino acids to build and repair your body*
- *To release your fat burning hormones*

30% Fat
- *To stabilize blood sugar and control hunger*
- *To provide essential fatty acids for hormone production*

Chapter Two

THE REAL POWER
OF FOODS

The real power of the Formula is the hormonal response generated from the foods you eat. Recent findings in dietary endocrinology (the hormonal effects of foods) have helped us understand the power of two hormones: insulin and glucagon. These two hormones are biological opposites. Think of insulin as a fat storing hormone and glucagon as a fat burning hormone. Now think of eating as a game. The object of the game is to eat a meal that controls the release of insulin and elevates glucagon. Do that and you win!

CONTROLLING INSULIN

High carbohydrate meals elevate blood sugar and stimulate the release of the hormone insulin. When blood sugar levels rise too high or too quickly, insulin's job is to siphon the excess into storage. Elevated insulin levels force the body to burn glucose for energy instead of stored body fat.

Insulin converts excess glucose into glycogen, removes it from the bloodstream, and stores it in your liver and muscle cells. Unfortunately, your body can store only small amounts of glycogen, and the excess glucose that your body can't store as glycogen will be converted into fat and stored in your fat cells.

When too much blood glucose is stored away, the brain is deprived of adequate amounts of its preferred fuel. The resulting low blood sugar triggers mood swings, hunger, and cravings for more carbohydrates. Over an extended period of time chronic elevated insulin levels can cause hypoglycemia or diabetes. Is it any wonder that diabetes is on the rise in this country, with all of the starchy and sugary carbohydrates that adults and children eat and drink?

With a better understanding of the negatives of high carbohydrate diets, one might question why we even eat carbohydrates.

Low carbohydrate diets can actually be worse than high carbohydrate diets because they deplete glucose and glycogen stores. Without glucose your body's only choice is to turn to stored fat and muscle mass to supply energy and attempt to control blood sugar. This produces the abnormal metabolic state called ketosis. When insufficient amounts of carbohydrates are eaten, the cells manufacture abnormal biochemicals known as ketone bodies. The idea is that if glucose is not an available source of energy, the body must burn fat for energy. Unfortunately, it's not quite that simple. When your body is in ketosis, yes, fat can be utilized for energy, but lean muscle mass and body proteins are also broken down and converted into glucose and used for energy as well. Sacrificing body proteins is the most inefficient way to supply glucose for your brain. Ketosis is not a healthy way to lose weight, not for one day, one week, or one month, and certainly not for the rest of your life.

Ketone bodies are actually waste products from incomplete fat metabolism and they accumulate in the blood. These toxic waste products make blood more acidic. The pH of the blood declines, upsetting the body's chemical balance, and excess ketone bodies spill into the urine. This can cause unpleasant side effects such as headaches, dizziness, fatigue, low blood sugar, muscle wasting, and nausea. The body attempts to get rid of ketone bodies through increased urination, so much of the actual weight loss is only water loss and can result in constipation. The water loss also leaches valuable electrolytes such as potassium from the bloodstream and can contribute to leg cramps and muscle fatigue.

But that's not the worst of it. Ketone bodies are also released through the lungs and can result in horrible body odor, bad breath, and a nasty taste in your mouth. I once spent three miserable hours on a plane next to a man who was in ketosis (I can smell a protein dieter before I see one). I've spoken with hundreds of people who call our hot line and listened to their horror stories about high protein dieting. Most of the people I have talked with have not enjoyed the side effects of eating the high protein diet at all.

ELEVATING GLUCAGON

A balanced meal helps stabilize blood sugar levels, controls insulin, and elevates the hormone glucagon. Glucagon will mobilize stored glycogen in the liver to maintain and balance blood sugar levels and allows stored body fat to be released and used as fuel.

Fat in a meal slows down the digestion and absorption of carbohydrates, so that glucose trickles gradually into the blood, providing the steady ongoing supply of glucose. The protein stimulates the release of the hormone glucagon, controlling insulin's effects and maintaining blood glucose concentrations within a normal range for a longer period of time. Glucagon also mobilizes the release of stored body fat from the adipose tissue (fat cells) directly into the bloodstream, allowing your muscle cells to burn fat, their preferred source of fuel, instead of glucose. The available glucose can be used by the brain to eliminate hunger and mood swings from meal to meal.

If protein stimulates the release of glucagon, the fat burning hormone, why not eat only protein? Once again, the high protein diet is not balanced and ketone bodies will form, along with all of their nasty side effects.

In addition to all of the horrible side effects of ketosis, new research indicates that ketogenic diets may cause permanent changes in fat cells, making them ten times more active in accumulating fat. When you begin eating carbohydrates again or go off your high protein diet, you gain weight at an alarming rate and often get fatter than you were before you started the diet. New evidence also indicates that continued ketosis leads to increased oxidation of lipids, an important factor in the development of heart disease. It's also known that excess calories from protein, fat, or carbohydrates will raise insulin levels. Finally, a lifetime of restricting carbohydrates is very unappetizing to people. Is a breakfast of eggs and bacon really good without toast and fruit? What's a deli sandwich without the bun? Pizza without the crust is just a mess. Before too long, you'll begin dreaming about green beans.

There's more than one way to achieve your weight loss goals. Instead of an extremely unbalanced diet, try the balanced 40-30-30 Formula approach. You will get all of the benefits of a high protein diet with none of the horrible side effects. The Formula offers a safe and balanced approach to fat burning and weight loss. Think about your entire family's eating habits, and you'll realize the Formula is for life.

SUMMARY

If the object of the game is to control insulin and elevate glucagon, simply learn how to eat balanced meals throughout the day. The Formula provides you with balanced meals in the revolutionary 40-30-30 ratio.

Chapter Three

THE 40-30-30 RATIO

Following the Formula is really quite simple. Every time you eat a meal or snack, have 40% of the total calories from carbohydrates, 30% from protein, and 30% from fat. Years of experience and working in our clinic with thousands of dieters taught us that most people aren't interested in how to figure the 40-30-30 caloric ratio; they just want to know what to eat and how much of it. Many people using the Formula look at the 40-30-30 Formula meals and haven't got a clue how we came up with the numbers. We don't think meals should be a math problem; in fact, that's precisely why we wrote this book. We did all of the work and the math for you. Simply follow the 21-Day Fat Flush Formula for three weeks and you will be an expert. But there are some people who want to understand how to determine the caloric ratio of a meal.

The 40-30-30 ratio is based on the calories of a meal. Since food manufacturers list carbohydrate, protein, and fat in grams on food labels, it can be difficult to determine the ratio of calories a food contains. Foods contain:

4 calories in one gram of carbohydrate

4 calories in one gram of protein

9 calories in one gram of fat

To determine the calories of a food, multiply the grams of carbohydrate and protein by 4 and fat grams by 9 and total them up. Then divide the carbohydrate calories by the total calories to determine the percentage of calories. Do the same with protein and fat.

To show you how to calculate the 40-30-30 ratio, I'll walk you through some samples.

Strawberry Smoothie

(from Fat Flush Formula breakfasts, plan C)

1⅔ cups fresh or frozen strawberries

¾   cup cold water

20 grams whey protein powder

1   tablespoon fructose

2⅓ tablespoons almonds

The nutritional profile of the Strawberry Smoothie, plan C, is:
Total Calories = 331   Carbohydrate = 33 grams, Protein = 25 grams, Fat = 11 grams

As previously mentioned, to determine the calories of a food, multiply the grams of carbohydrate and protein by 4, and the fat grams by 9 and total them up. Then divide the carbohydrate calories by the total calories to determine the percentage of calories. Do the same with protein and fat.

Strawberry Smoothie, plan C 40-30-30 ratio equals:

Carb. = 33 grams $\times 4 = 132$ carbohydrate calories

$132 \div 331$ total calories = 40% Carb.

Pro. = 25 grams $\times 4 = 100$ protein calories

$100 \div 331$ total calories = 30% Protein

Fat = 11 grams $\times 9 = 99$ fat calories

_____ $99 \div 331$ total calories = 30% Fat

331 = total calories

As you can see, the Strawberry Smoothie contains a perfect 40-30-30 ratio of carbohydrates, protein, and fat.

Cottage Cheese and Fruit

(from Fat Flush Formula breakfasts, plan B)

½   cup 2% lowfat cottage cheese

½   cup strawberries, sliced

½   kiwi, sliced

¼   cup grapes

2   teaspoons nuts

The nutritional profile of Cottage Cheese and Fruit, plan B, is:
Total Calories = 198   Carbohydrate = 20 grams, Protein = 16 grams, Fat = 6 grams

To determine the number of calories of a food, multiply the grams of carbohydrate and protein by 4 and fat grams by 9 and total them up. Then divide the carbohydrate calories by the total calories to determine the percentage of calories. Do the same with protein and fat.

Cottage Cheese and Fruit, plan B 40-30-30 ratio equals:

Carb. = 20 grams × 4 = 80 carbohydrate calories

$\qquad$ 80 ÷ 198 total calories = 40.3% Carb.

Pro. = 16 grams × 4 = 64 protein calories

$\qquad$ 64 ÷ 198 total calories = 32.3% Protein

Fat   = 6 grams   × 9 = 54 fat calories

$\qquad$ 54 ÷ 198 total calories = 27.3% Fat

198 = total calories

The Cottage Cheese and Fruit meal contains a 40-32-27 ratio of carbohydrate, protein, and fat. No, it's not exactly 40-30-30, but remember these next words: *Close is good enough.* Some meals will total 40-30-30 and others will be 41-31-28 or 42-29-29, or 39-32-29, etc. The point is, they all work! Foods vary, amounts vary. The meals don't have to be exact to work, and that's the beauty of the Formula. Close is good enough!

40-30-30 Nutrition Bar

(Balance Bar, Mocha flavor)

The nutritional profile of the 40-30-30 Nutrition Bar (Balance Bar, Mocha flavor) is:

Total Calories = 198   Carbohydrate = 22 grams, Protein = 14 grams, Fat = 6 grams

To determine the number of calories of the bar, multiply the grams of carbohydrate and protein by 4 and fat grams by 9 and total them up. Then divide the carbohydrate calories by the total calories to determine the percentage of calories. Do the same with protein and fat.

Carb. = 22 grams   × 4 =   88 carbohydrate calories

88 ÷ 198 total calories = 44.44% Carb.

Pro.   = 14 grams   × 4 =   56 protein calories

56 ÷ 198 total calories = 28.28% Protein

Fat   = 6 grams   × 9 =   54 fat calories

54 ÷ 198 total calories = 27.27% Fat

198 total calories

The Mocha Balance Bar contains an approximate 44-28-27 ratio of carbohydrate, protein, and fat. Now that you understand how to determine the 40-30-30 ratio of a meal, aren't you glad we did all the work for you? Practice with our meals. Choose your favorite meals and measure them out the first couple of times you make them so you have a good visual idea of your portion amounts. After that, you probably won't even need to measure. You will just know intuitively.

Chapter Four

RATING CARBOHYDRATES

I t is common knowledge that simple carbohydrates, such as sugar, are the dieter's downfall because they generate a surge in blood sugar and shortly thereafter a dramatic drop that leaves you sleepy, cranky, and craving more sugar. But we have been led to believe that complex carbohydrates such as bread and potatoes break down more slowly so the energy is released into the bloodstream in a flatter curve. However, since the introduction of the glycemic index, we know this view of the process is not really correct.

The glycemic index is a numerical system that rates how fast carbohydrate foods enter the bloodstream. In the early 1980s, the glycemic rating of carbohydrate foods was first introduced. At that time, glucose was thought to raise blood sugar the fastest and was rated 100. However, in 1990, additional foods were tested and many were found to be even higher. To make our point, we have broken down a small sample group of carbohydrate foods into the very high to very low range.

Very High Glycemic Index Foods (113–150)

Maltose (starch sugar)

Instant rice

Baked potato

Dates

Doughnuts

Most breakfast cereals

Pretzels

Rice cakes

Glucose (sugar)

High Glycemic Index Foods (76–112)

White bread

Honey

Raisins

Watermelon

Banana

Popcorn

Carrots

Rice

Corn

Medium Glycemic Index Foods (40–75)

Pasta al dente

Orange

Pear

Apple

Grapes

Sweet potato

Garbanzo beans

Low Glycemic Index Foods (0–39)

Milk

Oatmeal

Asparagus

Broccoli

Lentils

Grapefruit

Yogurt, plain

Barley

Fructose (fruit sugar)

Cherries

Nuts and seeds

From the above list, you will see that most breakfast cereals, pretzels, and rice cakes raise blood sugar more quickly than white bread. Raisins, popcorn, carrots, rice, and corn are all rated high. Most fruits and vegetables are medium to low glycemic. They are unprocessed, low in starch, and high in fiber. Fructose is a very low glycemic sweetener. It is actually sweeter than sugar, looks like granulated sugar, and can be found in most health food stores. We use it in place of sugar in many recipes, including our 40-30-30 Formula Desserts. Nuts are very low glycemic, since they contain carbohydrates along with protein and plenty of fat.

This list is not meant to have you completely avoid very high or high glycemic foods. The glycemic rating of a carbohydrate food is based on that food eaten alone. When carbohydrate foods are eaten together with protein and fat, the overall glycemic effect of that meal will be different. Protein and fat slow the digestion of carbohydrates so that glucose trickles into the bloodstream, lowering the glycemic response and keeping blood sugar levels steady. Therefore, white bread alone or bread with jelly would cause a substantial rise in blood glucose levels. But a sandwich consisting of white bread with sliced turkey, lettuce, tomato, and avocado will have a lower glycemic response, digest more slowly, and maintain steady blood sugar levels.

Most fruits, with the exception of bananas and dried fruits, are already low to medium glycemic. Fruit eaten with cottage cheese and nuts will have an even tighter control on blood glucose levels. Most fresh vegetables, with the exception of carrots, corn, and potatoes, are low to medium glycemic. Vegetables eaten with protein and fat will also allow tighter control of blood glucose levels. This is why we use primarily low to medium glycemic fruits and vegetables in the 21-Day Fat Flush Formula.

Isn't it interesting to note that breakfast cereals, baked potatoes, rice cakes, pretzels, pasta, bananas, and carrots are all high glycemic foods? Yet for years diet experts were promoting foods such as cereal with a banana for breakfast, a baked potato for lunch, a plate of pasta with red sauce for dinner, and rice cakes, carrot sticks, and pretzels for snacks. Is it any wonder these high-carbohydrate, low-fat diets didn't work?

The Formula incorporates the ultimate blend of carbohydrates, protein, and fat to help control blood glucose levels. We've done all of the work for you by taking into consideration the glycemic rating of carbohydrate foods when preparing Fat Flush Formula and Regular Formula Meals. Fat Flush

Formula meals contain only very low to medium rated glycemic carbohydrates for the tightest control of blood sugar levels. Regular Formula Meals provide an even greater variety of carbohydrate choices from low to high rated glycemic carbohydrates for continued weight loss or maintenance.

Refer to the Quick Reference Food Value and Glycemic Index Guide (page 277) for a list of glycemic rated foods.

Chapter Five

THE BENEFITS
OF EXERCISE

You've heard of the many benefits of exercise. Exercise burns calories, increases your metabolism, tones and builds muscle, and improves cardiovascular health and circulation. Exercise simply makes you feel better, healthier, and more fit. But the true power of exercise may actually lie in its hormonal effects. When you exercise, you lower insulin levels (the fat storing hormone), increase glucagon levels (the fat burning hormone), and release human growth hormone (HGH), the building and repairing hormone.

The effects of these powerful hormones can dramatically improve your ability to burn fat while you are losing weight and toning or building muscle.

One of the biggest misconceptions in sports nutrition is about what fuel source muscles prefer to use, glucose or fat. Most of the so-called experts will tell you it's glucose, but that is not true. New research has shown that muscles prefer to burn fat for energy, not glucose. Fat also provides a high-octane fuel supplying more than twice as much energy per gram as glucose. Fat contains 9 calories per gram while glucose contains only 4.

If you eat too many carbohydrates before exercise, blood sugar levels are spiked, stimulating the release of insulin, which forces your body to burn glucose for energy, preventing the release of stored body fat for most of the workout. But if you eat a balanced snack thirty minutes prior to exercise, blood sugar is balanced, releasing glucagon, which mobilizes stored body fat, maximizing your natural ability to burn fat for energy. If your diet is balanced and your blood sugar is stable before you begin your workout, you can burn fat as your primary source of energy during the entire workout and start to experience impressive results.

We worked with thousands of clients in our clinic, the BioSyn Human Performance Center in Kirkland, Washington, the world's first 40-30-30 zone nutrition clinic. It was located right next door to a large athletic club with more than 30,000 members. When we opened, I invited the aerobic instructors and private trainers over for a 40-30-30 nutrition presentation. At that time, everyone was eating a high carbohydrate diet, but we convinced the health club's staff to follow our diet plan for one month. It took only a few weeks before they saw dramatic changes in body fat levels, energy levels, and muscularity. They began referring hundreds of clients to us. But there is one woman we will never forget. Every evening she attended the 5:00 P.M. advanced aerobic class, six days a week. Each night at 4:55 P.M. we watched her walk into class eating a banana; then 60 minutes later she would leave drinking a high-carbohydrate sports drink. The trouble was her body never changed.

One day her aerobic instructor convinced her to stop by our clinic just to listen to what we had to say. She weighed 168 pounds and her body fat content was 38%—definitely too high given all the working out she was doing. Within 20 minutes of our explaining our program, she was in tears. We felt horrible and asked her what was the matter. She told us how frustrated she was. She had done everything her trainer told her to do: exercised six days a week, ate no fat and only carbohydrates, but she still had not lost any weight. She cried, "All my hard work and all I've been doing was burning banana!"

In as little as 20 minutes, she realized that all of the carbohydrates from the banana she ate each evening before her workout were causing her blood sugar levels to surge. Most of her workout was spent burning excess glucose from the banana rather than body fat. By the end of her workout, when her blood sugar levels were finally low enough to begin burning fat for energy, she drank a high-carbohydrate sports drink, and once again her blood sugar was spiked and insulin was released. The fat-storage, sugar-burning cycle was started all over again. She finally understood why she wasn't seeing any results from her workouts. She was actually sabotaging her workouts with a high-carbohydrate diet.

It didn't take long for her to see incredible results using the 40-30-30 Fat Flush Formula. She claimed her body began changing the next day simply by changing her pre- and post-workout snack. And it did. When the correct Formula of carbohydrates, protein, and fat enters the bloodstream, blood sugar is balanced, stimulating the production of glucagon—the body's natural fat burning hormone that burns fat and keeps energy levels and concentration high. Finally, your workouts begin to produce the kind of results you expect.

WHY EXERCISE?

We often get questions about exercise. The three most common are as follows:

1. *Do I have to exercise to get results on the Formula?* The answer is no. You don't *have* to exercise to see results on the Formula, but everyone *should* exercise. We have worked with hundreds of people who either chose not to exercise or for health reasons could not exercise but still lost weight and had increased energy levels. However, even though you do not have to exercise to benefit from the Formula, we highly recommend it. With even just a little exercise you can experience even better results.

2. *How much exercise should I do?* Experts recommend exercising three to five days per week for 20 to 60 minutes at a time for best results. There is really no right or wrong amount of time that you should exercise, although too much exercise or overtraining is not good. Studies have shown that some exercise improves immune response, but too much suppresses immune response. It is recommended to exercise enough to achieve these three components of fitness: cardiovascular endurance, strength and muscular endurance, and flexibility. It's probably best to think of the Nike slogan and "Just do it."

3. *What type of exercise is best?* Research shows that you should combine aerobic and anaerobic exercise with stretching to gain the best results from exercise.

Aerobic exercise increases your cardiovascular endurance. Aerobic exercises include swimming, brisk walking, jogging, fast bicycling, aerobic dance, stationary machines such as treadmills, skiing, and sports such as tennis (singles), soccer, hockey, and basketball.

Anaerobic exercise develops strength and increases muscular endurance. Anaerobic exercise involves weight resistance using either your own body weight in exercises such as push-ups or squats, or dumbbells, free weights, and/or exercise machines.

Stretching promotes flexibility. All of us should include stretching in our exercise programs. Recent studies have shown that it is best to stretch after exercise, when your muscles are warmer and less vulnerable to injury. Stretching reduces soreness and increases strength and flexibility while it relaxes the muscles you just used. It also increases joint range of motion and reduces the risk of muscle strains, tears, and ruptures. Stretching is particularly important as you age for strengthening tendons.

THE 40-30-30 EXERCISE FORMULA

We have developed a new approach to exercise called the 40-30-30-Exercise Formula. It's easy and fun, and anyone can do it. No matter what your training, start by determining how much time you can devote to your workout and what your exercise focus is. If your present workout consists primarily of aerobic exercise, spend 40% of your workout doing aerobic exercise, 30% doing anaerobic exercise, and 30% stretching. However, if your focus is on building muscle, spend 40% of your workout on anaerobic exercise, 30% on aerobic exercise, and 30% on stretching.

SAMPLE EXERCISE PLANS

The following are sample plans for those whose focus is on aerobic exercise. Any forms of aerobic and anaerobic exercise may be used. Those listed are only examples. Start with an activity you find comfortable. When you feel it is time to progress to a more challenging level, increase the overall time and intensity of your workout.

BEGINNER EXAMPLE

If you are exercising at a beginner level, 20 minutes a day for three to five days a week is a good goal. Spend eight minutes fast walking (aerobic), six minutes doing upper-body weight training (anaerobic), and six minutes stretching. Upper-body weight training can be as simple as arm curls and front and side arm raises holding a can of soup in each hand or light hand weights (two to three pounds).

BEGINNER/INTERMEDIATE EXAMPLE

If you are exercising at a beginner/intermediate level, 40 minutes a day for four to five days a week is a good goal. Spend 16 minutes fast walking, swimming, or fast stationary bicycling (aerobic); 12 minutes lifting weights or using weight machines (anaerobic); and 12 minutes stretching.

INTERMEDIATE EXAMPLE

If you are exercising at an intermediate level, 50 minutes a day for five days per week is a good goal. Spend 20 minutes fast walking or jogging, swimming, or using indoor stationary machines (aerobic); 15 minutes lifting free weights, using weight machines, or doing push-ups and lunges (anaerobic); and 15 minutes stretching.

INTERMEDIATE/ADVANCED EXAMPLE

If you are exercising at an intermediate/advanced level, 60 minutes a day for five days per week is a good goal. Spend 24 minutes running, swimming, or using high intensity indoor stationary machines (aerobic); 18 minutes lifting free weights, using weight machines, or doing push-ups and lunges (anaerobic); and 18 minutes of stretching.

Consult your doctor prior to embarking on significant lifestyle changes. He or she can establish your initial state of health and advise you as to any personal concerns you should have while making changes in exercise and diet.

Chapter Six

THE FORMULA IS NOT
JUST FOR LOSING WEIGHT

The Formula is a personalized, balanced nutrition program that provides a preventive approach for a lifetime. The health benefits of balanced nutrition have been well established. Why take drugs to prevent your risk of disease when you can use balanced nutrition with none of the side effects?

It's well documented that elevated insulin levels are now being directly linked to many diseases such as hypertension, hyperlipidemia, type II diabetes, and obesity. Elevated insulin levels are primarily caused by an unbalanced diet. The Formula gives you the power to take control of insulin levels with the foods you eat. It becomes your direct link to longevity. The Formula provides the solution to living a healthy life and feeling the best you can feel.

Over the years, we have worked with hundreds of doctors and heard from thousands of people who have improved their lives by using the 40-30-30 Formula.

IMPROVED BRAIN FUNCTION

Your brain requires a steady supply of glucose. When blood sugar levels are out of balance, concentration suffers and overall brain function is decreased.

The Formula can help keep blood sugar balanced. We have heard numerous testimonials through the years. One of our favorites was about a little girl whose entire family began using the Formula and enjoyed its many benefits. One morning they woke up late for school and had to rush to make the bus. As the mom took a deep breath and watched the bus drive away, she noticed the brake lights come on and the bus stop. Her daughter came flying out of the bus, yelling, "Mom, I forgot my bar and my brain can't think without it." Mom had switched the family from pastries and cereal for breakfast to eating a 40-30-30 Nutrition Bar instead, and the little girl had started to feel much better.

By correcting blood sugar imbalances, the Formula helps stabilize blood sugar levels and improves overall concentration and brain clarity.

MENTAL HEALTH

To maintain proper mental health, it is critical that your diet provide adequate amounts of protein. Protein supplies amino acids, which are the building blocks for your brain's powerful neurotransmitters.

We have spoken with numerous psychiatrists and psychologists who have noticed remarkable improvements in their patients' mental health when they followed the 40-30-30 Formula nutrition program.

IMPROVING SLEEP

Hundreds of people through the years have commented on how the 40-30-30 ratio has also improved their sleep. They sleep more soundly and actually wake more easily, feeling rested and alert. A retired man said to us that he was waking earlier, refreshed and ready to go. Now he had too much time on his hands! A woman told me that her husband was no longer grumpy in the morning and began calling himself a morning person. She claims he never had been before.

Many people experience difficulty falling asleep or staying asleep, or wake up feeling groggy after eating high carbohydrate snacks before bed. High carb meals or snacks cause blood sugar and insulin levels to rise. These imbalances can disrupt sleep patterns. The Formula can help keep blood sugar balanced and thereby improve sleep.

FEMALE HORMONES

Women who crave carbohydrates before and during their menstrual cycle or who suffer from mood swings, headaches, cramps, and water retention should take a look at their diets.

We have heard from many women that after they use the Formula 40-30-30 nutrition program, their cravings for carbohydrates decline and many, if not all, of their PMS symptoms disappear. One woman commented that she wasn't even aware that her period was starting because she wasn't retaining fluids, didn't crave chocolate, and had no headaches or cramps. Her family noticed how pleasant she had become. She called us to make sure she would always stay that way. We told her she would turn back into that bloated, miserable crab only if she went back to her old eating habits!

We've worked with many Ob/Gyns who recommend the Formula to their patients who suffer from hot flashes and hormonal imbalances. In fact, one Ob/Gyn in San Diego encourages every one of his patients to follow the 40-30-30 nutrition program.

For many women, the Formula is the powerful first step needed to maintain blood sugar and insulin levels and help balance female hormones.

DIABETES

With diabetes on the rise, almost every pharmaceutical manufacturer is producing treatments in the form of pills and easy-to-use injection pens. One of the top pharmaceutical companies has built the largest factory ever, dedicated to the production of a single drug—insulin. However, in a recent report in *The New England Journal of Medicine*, scientists note that controlling dietary carbohydrates and fiber had the same effect on blood glucose levels as drugs to control blood sugar levels.

We've had many reports from diabetics who were able to reduce their use of insulin and pills by 50% or more. One woman sent me a note that she had been using 110 units of insulin per day and three drugs. After using the Formula, she was able to drop her use of insulin down to 10 units and one pill per day and said she feels human again.

The Formula is designed to help keep blood sugar levels steady, thereby helping to control the body's demand for insulin. This not only helps diabetics in controlling their blood sugar naturally, it can help to reduce the risk of diabetes for others.

HYPOGLYCEMIA

Hypoglycemia is a reaction to eating too many carbohydrates at a meal. Blood sugar levels surge, and insulin is elevated to reduce them. But for many people, blood sugar drops too low and hypoglycemic symptoms start to set in.

Joyce can speak firsthand about hypoglycemia. For years she followed a high-carbohydrate diet and suffered from blood sugar crashes almost daily at 11:00 A.M. and 3:00 P.M. It took literally one day of the 40-30-30 Formula's caloric ratio to convince her that we had stumbled onto one of the greatest breakthroughs ever in nutrition. The Formula can keep blood sugar levels balanced from meal to meal, thus helping to avoid hypoglycemia.

HIGH BLOOD PRESSURE

High blood glucose levels stimulate the release of insulin. Elevated insulin levels cause negative hormone reactions that can lead to the constriction of blood vessels and thereby increase blood pressure.

One of our clients told us that she had been taking medication to lower her blood pressure and began using the Formula on her doctor's recommendation. Thirty days later she returned to her doctor. When she called to report the good news, we enjoyed hearing her doctor's explanation that she never really needed medication; she simply needed a balanced diet.

The Formula helps keep blood sugar balanced, controlling the release of insulin, thereby triggering positive hormonal reactions that further control insulin and can help promote vasodilation, actually widening blood vessels and reducing blood pressure.

HIGH CHOLESTEROL

High cholesterol has been linked to high levels of insulin (hyperinsulinism). Hyperinsulinemia stimulates an enzyme (HMG CoA) in the body that increases the liver's production of cholesterol. By controlling insulin, you control the release of this enzyme and lower cholesterol levels.

We spoke with a man who told us he tried to lower his cholesterol for months by watching his diet. His doctor told him to cut out all fatty foods and eat lots of carbohydrates. For two months he cut out all eggs, red meat, and dairy. He even began pouring fruit juice on his cereal each morning in place of milk. To his horror, when he went back to his doctor, he found his cholesterol levels had skyrocketed along with his weight. His doctor immediately put him on a drug to lower his high levels of cholesterol.

A nurse in the office overheard the man's complaints and told him about the Formula she and her husband were following with great results. He bought the book that day. Thirty days later he returned for a follow-up visit. He had lost 22 pounds and his cholesterol had dropped so dramatically that the doctor took him off the drug and encouraged him to follow the diet for the rest of his life.

DEFENSIVE NUTRITION

It makes sense to believe that you are what you eat. Many people with poor diets suffer from weak immune systems. Poorly balanced diets stimulate negative hormonal reactions in the body that weaken the immune system, increasing susceptibility to illness and disease. A balanced diet strengthens the immune system and acts as a defensive nutrition insurance policy to protect you from disease.

HYPERACTIVITY

Childhood obesity has doubled in the last ten years, and it is reported that only 10% of children get even the minimum RDA of vitamins and minerals. And of course many kids are picky eaters. Many kids love junk food and suffer from mood swings and behavioral problems; they also have poor immune response. To make matters worse, the drug companies respond with powerful mood-altering drugs.

We have seen that many hyperactive kids are eating high carbohydrate diets that are far too low in protein. High carbohydrate diets spike blood sugar levels, and insulin levels rise in an attempt to lower them. If their blood sugar drops too low, children get cranky and experience symptoms of hunger, loss of concentration, and poor performance. High carbohydrate diets are also low in protein. Protein provides the amino acids needed for building healthy strong bodies and balancing brain chemistry.

The Formula contains kids' favorite meals that can help balance blood sugar levels; provide amino acids, fatty acids, and adequate glucose for the brain; help improve focus and concentration; and control hunger and mood swings.

We have heard from many parents who report that their children's moods and behavior dramatically improved when they changed their diets and began following the 40-30-30 Formula.

CHILDHOOD OBESITY

According to recent studies, 25% of Americans under the age of nineteen are now overweight or obese. American teens spend more than five hours a day in front of some kind of screen, be it TV or computer. Inactivity and high carbohydrate junk-food diets are the main culprits. With french fries and potato chips listed as kids' most popular vegetable, is it any wonder new cases of type II diabetes in children are at an all-time high?

One of the most rewarding phone calls we ever got came from a woman who told us about her twelve-year-old son, who weighed 165 pounds. His first day back at school was devastating and he informed his mother that he didn't want to go back because all of the kids made fun of him. His mother had recently attended a seminar we presented and she had asked her son to read our book, *40-30-30 Fat Burning Nutrition*. He read the book and said, "Mom, I can do this." They worked together to follow the 40-30-30 meals, and for the first time in his life he began to see the scale go down. *The Formula is not just for adults; everyone can benefit from balanced nutrition, especially children.*

BUILDING MUSCLE

Although millions of people struggle with losing weight, some individuals have difficulty putting muscle on. It seems that no matter what they eat, they are skinny as a rail. We've worked with teenage boys and all types of athletes who were consuming 5,000 calories or more per day. They lifted weights but were still unable to gain muscle mass.

The Formula works to increase lean muscle mass by providing adequate amounts of carbohydrate, protein, and fat. Blood sugar levels stabilize, controlling insulin and elevating glucagon. Strength training stimulates the release of human growth hormone. With the release of glucagon and human growth hormone, the body can begin to build lean muscle mass.

Through the years we have heard from thousands of athletes who have given up their high carbohydrate diets and now swear by the 40-30-30 Formula. They have gained lean muscle mass, decreased body fat, increased recovery rates, reduced lactic acid buildup, and improved overall performance.

Chapter Seven

WHY MOST WEIGHT LOSS PROGRAMS FAIL

For years there have been hundreds of diets that promise weight loss. While there are many reasons why diets fail, the most obvious are listed below.

1. Most diets are not balanced.

They recommend foods that stimulate the wrong hormonal reaction to burn fat and lose weight. Every time you eat, the balance of the carbohydrates, protein, and fat in the meal combines to regulate the hormones that burn fat or store fat in your body.

2. Most diets are not personalized.

They use a one-size-fits-all concept. We are all unique individuals with our own unique nutritional requirements. A diet that does not specify portion control and allows you to eat as much or as little as you want fails to take into consideration your specific requirements.

3. Most diets are not easy.

They are far too restrictive and difficult to follow, and certainly not something you can employ for a lifetime. For any diet or nutrition program to be successful, it should be easy to follow and should provide detailed meal plans that show you exactly what to eat. It has to have appealing foods, it needs to make sense, and it should be one that your entire family can use.

COMPARING DIFFERENT DIETS

Through the years we have helped thousands of people use the 40-30-30 Formula. We have worked with all types of people who have come to us after failing on just about every type of diet known. To help you further understand how the Formula works and why most diets fail, we have described the most popular diets and some of the reasons why they don't work.

HIGH PROTEIN DIETS

High protein diets encourage you to eat primarily protein, restricting your intake of carbohydrates. Although many people experience weight loss, the side effects are many and the long-term results are dismal. Here are just a few of the reasons why high protein diets are bound to fail:

• High protein diets are too low in carbohydrates. Any diet that provides less than 100 grams of carbohydrates per day can cause blood sugar imbalances and low blood sugar. Consuming too few carbohydrates causes ketosis, which can cause you to lose muscle. Losing muscle is the worst thing you can do because it slows your metabolism. As your metabolism slows, your body burns fewer calories and less fat. Ketosis also causes horrible body odor and bad breath from the ketone gas that oozes out of your body.

• High protein diets are far too high in protein and fat. Besides not being balanced, high protein diets fail to teach portion control and allow you to eat as much protein as you want, which can also contain excess fat. But excess protein calories are converted into and stored as fat. Also, a little-known fact is that excess protein and fat calories can also stimulate the fat storage hormone insulin, just the same as excess carbohydrates can.

• High protein diets are far too restrictive and difficult to follow. After only a few days of gorging on fatty meats, you'll begin dreaming of forbidden carbohydrates. High protein diets can be very difficult to follow and are certainly not a diet that your entire family can use.

LOWFAT DIETS

Lowfat diets usually encourage you to eat as many lowfat or fatfree carbohydrates as you want and restrict eating adequate amounts of healthy protein and fat. They can also be referred to as high carbohydrate diets. Here are just a few of the reasons why lowfat/high carbohydrate diets are bound to fail:

• Lowfat/high carbohydrate diets are far too high in carbohydrates. Very popular in the 1980s, these diets have been proven to fail, since too many carbohydrates in a meal can spike blood sugar levels and elevate the fat storing hormone insulin. High insulin prevents you from burning fat efficiently. Besides not being balanced, high carbohydrate diets don't teach portion control and leave you craving more carbohydrates and feeling hungry all the time.

• Lowfat/high carbohydrate diets provide inadequate amounts of protein. If you do not get enough high quality protein, or more important, the right ratio of amino acids that are found in high quality protein, you will lose muscle mass and other critical body proteins. When muscle is lost, your metabolism slows and your body burns fewer calories and less fat.

• Lowfat/high carbohydrate diets are deficient in essential fats. High carbohydrate diets restrict fat, which can leave you feeling hungry all the time. That's why they suggest you eat every two hours. Essential fatty acid deficiency can also cause hormonal imbalances.

• High carbohydrate diets are far too restrictive and difficult to follow. By restricting many types of healthy proteins and fats, high carbohydrate, lowfat diets can be very bland, boring, and difficult to follow. Try getting your family to eat fat-free veggie burgers and rice cakes every day.

VERY LOW CALORIE DIETS

Very low calorie diets have been proven not to work. Low calorie diets should be done under medical supervision and are generally short term, as their side effects can be severe. They generally consist of a drink mix available by prescription only. Here are just a few of the reasons why very low calorie diets are bound to fail:

• Very low calorie diets are too low in essential fats. You need fat to stay healthy as well as to actually help you burn fat. Inadequate fat in your diet can cause you to be hungry all the time and can lead to blood sugar imbalances, dry skin and hair, and hormone imbalances.

• Lowfat, low calorie diets are far too low in quality protein. Inadequate protein in your diet contributes to muscle breakdown and amino acid deficiencies and slows your metabolism. As your metabolism declines, your body burns fewer calories and less fat.

• Very low calorie diets contain too little carbohydrate, causing ketosis to develop. Lean body tissues are lost and dehydration occurs.

• Very low calorie diets teach dangerous eating habits by relying on extreme measures. When you return to eating a mixed diet, dramatic fluid retention and swelling generally occur, with rapid weight gain. Very low calorie diets fail to teach portion control and are certainly not designed for a lifetime.

FOOD COMBINING DIETS

Food combining diet plans restrict you from eating certain foods together. They promote only fruit for breakfast and restrict you from eating many carbohydrates and proteins together. Here are just a few of the reasons why these types of diets are bound to fail:

• Food combining diets can be too high in carbohydrates. If breakfast consists only of fruit, blood sugar can surge, stimulating the release of insulin to lower it. Elevated insulin prevents you from burning fat efficiently.

• Food combining diets can be too low in protein. Without adequate protein in your meals (especially for breakfast), you can lose muscle, as well as decrease the fat burning hormone glucagon. Losing muscle slows your metabolism. As your metabolism declines, your body burns fewer calories and less fat for energy.

• Food combining diets do not teach portion control. These diets typically allow you to eat as much as you want as long as you are following the arcane food combining rules. Excess calories, regardless of any type of combining rules, will be converted into fat, which is stored in your fat cells. Excess calories also stimulate the release of the fat storing hormone insulin.

• Food combining diets are way too restrictive and difficult to follow. The combining rules are hard to follow, which causes most dieters to simply give up. If you have been following food combining in an attempt to improve digestion, you are going about it the wrong way. Poor digestion is due to a lack of digestive enzymes. A balanced diet, with adequate amounts of protein supplying the amino acids that build your digestive enzymes, is a much better approach to correcting poor digestion.

NO-SUGAR DIETS

No-sugar diets restrict you from eating any type of sugar or "white" foods and allow you to eat only their "acceptable foods." Here are just a few of the reasons why no-sugar diets are bound to fail:

• No-sugar diets can be unbalanced and too low in carbohydrates. Many of the recommended meals are simply not balanced. When analyzed, they are no different from high protein, low carbohydrate diets, and you can experience all of the same problems that those diets have.

• No-sugar diets are one-size-fits-all diets. Their simplistic mantra fails to teach portion control. Eating too many or too few calories will cause poor results.

• No-sugar diets are far too restrictive and difficult to follow. Compulsive, restrictive diets are bound to fail. In reality, there is nothing wrong with sugar, sweet foods, or "white" foods. A balanced meal should contain carbohydrates, protein, and fats to stabilize blood sugar levels and balance hormonal reactions from meal to meal.

VEGETARIAN DIETS

Vegetarian diets restrict the consumption of animal products and tell you to eat as many plant-based foods as you want. There are three main types of vegetarian diets:

• Vegan or strict vegetarian diets eliminate all animal products.

• Lacto vegetarian diets eliminate meat and fish but allow dairy products.

• Ovo-lacto vegetarian diets eliminate meat and fish but allow dairy and egg products.

We recommend the lacto or ovo-lacto vegetarian diet for those following a vegetarian diet. They are less restrictive, so it is easier to get adequate amounts of high quality protein. Many of the meals found in the Formula conform to vegetarian guidelines. If you are a vegetarian, you can alter any meals containing objectionable protein sources and substitute lowfat tofu or tempeh. Here are just a few of the reasons why restrictive vegetarian diets can fail:

• Vegetarian diets can be too high in carbohydrates. Too many carbohydrates can elevate blood sugar levels and stimulate the fat storing hormone insulin. Vegetarian diets seldom teach portion control and usually allow you to eat as many carbohydrates as you want.

• Vegetarian diets can be too low in high quality, easy-to-digest proteins. If you do not get enough high quality protein, or more significant, the ratio of amino acids that are found in high quality protein, you can lose muscle and tear down other body proteins. Lysine deficiencies are commonly seen in vegans. Many vegetarians believe that combining beans and rice provides a complete protein. First of all, beans and rice are primarily carbohydrates. They provide a very small amount of protein, each containing certain amino acids the other may be lacking. When combined, the small amount of protein they contain may be complete, but it is certainly not providing adequate amounts of quality protein to build and repair a healthy body. That explains why so many vegetarians we have worked with through the years have had such high percentages of body fat. Even thin vegetarians had high percentages of body fat. Unfortunately, they were losing too much lean muscle mass.

• Vegetarian diets can be restrictive and difficult to follow. By restricting many types of healthy proteins, high carbohydrate vegan diets can be very bland, boring, and difficult to follow. Try getting your family to eat veggie burgers and tofu hot dogs.

RAW FOOD DIETS

Raw food diets usually allow you to eat anything you want as long as it is not cooked. Raw food diets are usually vegan diets (strict vegetarians). Here are just a few of the reasons why these types of diets are bound to fail:

• Raw food diets can be high in carbohydrates. They restrict you from eating most animal protein and contain primarily carbohydrates.

• Raw food diets can be too low in protein. Most animal protein foods require cooking or some type of processing. If you do not get enough protein in your meals you can lose muscle, as well as decrease glucagon, the fat burning hormone, and slow your metabolism. As your metabolism declines, your body burns fewer calories and less fat.

• Raw food diets do not teach portion control. These diets typically allow you to eat as much as you want as long as you are eating raw food. Excess calories from any kind of food, raw or not, will be converted into fat and stored in your fat cells. Excess calories can also stimulate the production of the fat storing hormone insulin.

• Raw food diets are far too restrictive and tedious to follow. Also, eating excessively large amounts of nuts and seeds can cause amino acid imbalances, leading to viral outbreaks.

DIET PATCHES, HERBAL PILLS, AND DIET PILLS

Diet patches and herbal and diet pill programs allow you to eat anything you want and try to make you believe that some special patch, pill, or herbal mix will increase your metabolism so you lose all the weight you want. Many patches and diet pills have serious side effects, can be highly addictive, and can affect the heart and central nervous system. Others are completely worthless. Here are just a few of the reasons why diet patches and pills are bound to fail.

• Patches and diet pills are usually loaded with stimulants and appetite suppressants that can reduce hunger. Without food, your body thinks it's starving and reserves its fat. The resulting weight loss is primarily muscle and water weight, with very little fat loss. By not eating adequate calories for your size and activity level, you will experience all of the problems associated with a very low calorie diet. You need to eat to maximize fat burning and spare lean muscle mass. Remember, not only do you lose muscle mass in your arms and legs, you are also losing it in your heart.

• Patches and diet pill programs do not teach portion control. In fact, some encourage you to eat anything you want as long as you are taking the magic pills. Excess calories from any meal will be converted into fat and stored in your fat cells.

• Patches and diet pills do not teach you good eating habits. The most powerful thing you can do to increase your metabolism and burn fat is to eat balanced meals based on your particular carbohydrate, protein, and fat requirements.

FAT AND STARCH BLOCKERS

The developers of pills that block fat or starch from your diet encourage you to rely on those pills to eliminate excess fat and starch from your diet. Here are just a few of the reasons why fat and starch blockers are bound to fail.

• Fat and starch blockers can cause nutritional and hormonal imbalances. Fat blockers cannot differentiate between good and bad fats. Dieters will generally eat more saturated fat in a meal, relying on the fat blocker to eliminate it. The sad fact is that by blocking the absorption of good fat, essential fatty acid deficiencies can occur. You also get to deal with the oily discharge that can leak out of your body.

• Fat and starch blockers do not teach portion control. These diets can encourage you to eat as much as you want as long as you are taking the magic pills. Excess calories from any meal, whether they are from carbohydrates, protein, or fat, will be converted into fat and stored in your fat cells.

• Fat and starch blockers do not teach you good eating habits. The most powerful thing you can do to increase your metabolism and burn fat is to learn how to eat a balanced diet that stabilizes blood sugar for proper hormone regulation.

MOST OTHER FAD DIETS

Almost any type of diet falls into one of the above categories. So simply remember, when choosing a diet and nutrition program, to make sure that it is balanced with carbohydrates, protein, and fat at every meal, is personalized for your specific size and level of activity, and is easy enough to follow for the rest of your life. Don't follow any diet that you wouldn't want your entire family to use.

THE FORMULA

The Formula is not really a diet but a balanced eating plan for you and your family to follow for life. The Formula may take some effort at first, but it is not complicated. It teaches you how to eat the balanced 40-30-30 nutrition ratio at every meal. Unlike any other diet and nutrition program that has ever been developed, the Formula provides you with detailed A, B, C, D, and E personalized meal planners, each suited for your personal requirements. The Formula is so easy that anyone can use it.

- **The Formula is balanced.**

    The Formula uses the revolutionary 40-30-30 nutrition ratio at every meal and snack. The 40-30-30 nutrition ratio recommends that 40% of the total calories come from carbohydrates, 30% from protein, and 30% from fats. Balanced nutrition and blood sugar control are two of the main reasons why the Formula works so well.

- **The Formula is personalized.**

    The Formula is a nutrition program that is personalized for your individual

> ### A Healthy Diet Plan
> - *Balanced with carbohydrates, protein, and fat*
> - *Personalized for your specific size and level of activity*
> - *Easy to use*
> - *Suitable for your entire family*

requirements. This is yet another reason why the Formula works so well. Unlike any other diet program or nutrition book that has ever been written, the Formula provides five distinct meal plans that have been painstakingly personalized to fit your individual requirements. We did all the hard work for you. More important, this personalized approach teaches you portion control to enhance fat loss. Too much food will slow weight loss, but too little food will slow your metabolism and just as easily inhibit fat loss. Adequate calories are vital for weight loss and longevity.

• **The Formula is easy and tells you exactly what to do.**

The Formula is like having your own personal nutrition coach helping you reach your goals. The complete nutrition program gives you everything you need and tells you exactly how to do it. And because the Formula uses the revolutionary 40-30-30 balanced nutrition ratio, no food is really off-limits when used in moderation and in the proper ratio.

Part Two

THE 21-DAY
FAT FLUSH PROGRAM

Chapter Eight

GETTING STARTED

For the next 21 days, you will be following what we refer to as the Fat Flush Formula. If you have been following a very high carbohydrate diet, eating lots of sugar or very little protein, please use one week of our Regular Formula Meals before beginning the 21-Day Fat Flush Formula.

We originally developed the Fat Flush Plan for athletes who needed to get "shredded." This is a term made popular in bodybuilding, referring to the appearance of athletes' muscle tissue containing very low body fat. For six weeks prior to competition, an athlete would follow the Fat Flush Plan. He would lose body fat without sacrificing any lean muscle mass and continue to gain muscle. In just six weeks, he would get in contest shape. The results were so impressive, we developed a less restrictive plan for our average clients. Our first book, *40-30-30 Fat Burning Nutrition,* contained only one week of Fat Flush meals. We heard from thousands of our readers requesting more Fat Flush meals. Our years of trial and error have resulted in the 21-Day Fat Flush Formula.

We have included a wide variety of foods to choose from, including family style meals, kids' favorites, and even desserts. After using the 21-Day Fat Flush Formula for the full three weeks, you may decide to continue using Fat Flush meals until you reach your goal weight or use them in conjunction with the Regular Meals. Many of our clients use Fat Flush meals exclusively. Since 1991, we have been using a combination of both. The choice is yours.

We always remind our clients to keep it simple. Begin using the 21-Day Fat Flush Formula by finding a few breakfasts, a few lunches, and some snacks you like and learn how to make those right for your personal requirements. There are many choices for dinners, including family style meals and kids' favorites your whole family will enjoy.

By no means should you feel that you must prepare every one of the Fat Flush Formula meals. Use the meals you like and you will get the best results. It doesn't matter if you eat the same few meals every day for the rest of your life. Think about it—many people have been eating the same bowl of cereal and glass of juice every day of their lives. Doesn't it make sense to learn how to make a balanced breakfast and switch to that instead? We eat a 40-30-30 Nutrition Bar or shake almost every morning with tea, coffee, or water. It's easy, we like it, and it makes us feel great for the next four hours.

FIVE EASY STEPS TO SUCCESS

One of the reasons the Formula works so well is that it is a complete and personalized nutrition program. Unlike any other diet or nutrition book ever written, we have created five different meal plans, one of which will provide your personal requirements based on your gender, size, and activity level. The Formula works because it is not a one-size-fits-all program and because the meals you choose contain the right proportion of carbohydrates, protein, and fats to unleash your body's powerful fat burning potential. In fact, when you eat the 40-30-30 Formula of carbohydrates, protein, and fats, your body has no choice but to burn fat for energy.

To make it as easy as possible for you to succeed, begin by following these five easy steps:

1. Know your requirements.

Choose the correct meal plan for your personal requirements from the Formula Meal Plan Selection Chart (page 63).

2. Choose your favorite meals.

Review all of the Fat Flush Formula Meals and choose several from breakfast, lunch, snacks, and dinner that sound good to you.

3. Go shopping.

Refer to the Formula Shopping Guide (page 285) to prepare a shopping list. Go shopping for everything you will need. It is also a good idea to get rid of all of the junk food that you have around so that you will not be tempted.

4. Follow the 21-Day Fat Flush Program.

Don't wait to get started until Monday. Begin today at your very next meal. You will be amazed at the results you are going to get in as little as 21 days if you follow the program as closely as possible. Don't try to make your own meals until you have followed the 21-Day Fat Flush Program. When designing your own meals becomes a math problem, many people become frustrated and give up, so don't try to do it yourself in the beginning. Let us be your nutrition coach for the next 21 days.

5. Monitor your results.

Use the Star Tracker Nutrition Journal and the Monthly Tracker guides to monitor your success.

WHAT MEAL PLAN
IS RIGHT FOR YOU?

The Formula personalized meal plans have been designed for your individual 40-30-30 requirements. Your gender, body weight, and activity level determine the overall amount of food and number of calories you need daily to maximize the burning of stored fat for energy. There are five different plans for you to choose from.

When choosing the plan, use your current actual weight, not your goal weight. For example, if you are a woman weighing 195 pounds and moderately active, choose the C plan. When your weight drops to 180 pounds, switch to the B plan.

Review the Formula Meal Plan Selection Chart on the next page to choose the correct plan for your requirements.

If you are an elite athlete training more than ten hours per week and competitive in your sport, you will certainly require more calories than a noncompetitive person the same size. Highly trained muscles have greater energy requirements. Review the Formula Meal Plan Selection Chart for Elite Athletes (page 64) to choose the correct size plan for your needs.

THE FORMULA
MEAL PLAN SELECTION CHART

WOMEN

Activity Level	Low–Moderate	Medium–High
Hours of Exercise per Week	Exercise 0–4 hours per week	Exercise 5–10 hours per week
Current Body Weight	*Use Meal Planner*	*Use Meal Planner*
Under 140	A	B
141–180	B	C
181–200+	C	D

MEN

Activity Level	Low–Moderate	Medium–High
Hours of Exercise per Week	Exercise 0–4 hours per week	Exercise 5–10 hours per week
Current Body Weight	*Use Meal Planner*	*Use Meal Planner*
Under 140	B	C
141–180	C	D
181–250+	C	D

Your Personalized Meal Plan is _____

THE FORMULA
MEAL PLAN SELECTION CHART FOR ELITE ATHLETES

FEMALE ELITE ATHLETES

Current Body Weight	Train 10 or more hours per week
Under 140	C
141–180	D
180 and over	E

MALE ELITE ATHLETES

Current Body Weight	Train 10 or more hours per week
Under 140	C
141–180	D
180 and over	E

MACRONUTRIENT CHART

Listed below are the total grams of carbohydrates, protein, fat, and calories listed for each meal plan. The meal plans have been tailored for individual requirements based on gender, weight, and activity levels. To determine which meal plan is right for you, refer to the Formula Meal Plan Selection Chart. Each meal and snack contains the 40-30-30 ratio, which provides 40% of its total calories from carbohydrate, 30% from protein, and 30% from fat.

Personal Meal Plan	A	B	C	D	E
BREAKFAST					
Carbohydrate grams	20	20	33	47	53
Protein grams	15	15	25	35	40
Fat grams	6	6	11	13	18
Calories	194	194	331	445	534
LUNCH					
Carbohydrate grams	27	40	40	53	66
Protein grams	20	30	30	40	50
Fat grams	9	14	14	18	22
Calories	269	406	406	534	662
SNACKS					
Carbohydrate grams	20	20	20	20	40
Protein grams	15	15	15	15	30
Fat grams	6	6	6	6	12
Calories	194	194	194	194	388
DINNER					
Carbohydrate grams	40	47	53	53	66
Protein grams	30	35	40	40	50
Fat grams	14	15	18	18	22
Calories	406	463	534	534	662

Personal Meal Plan	A	B	C	D	E
DAILY TOTALS					
Carbohydrate grams	106	126	146	173	226
Protein grams	80	95	110	130	170
Fat grams	35	42	48	57	75
Calories	1,063	1,257	1,465	1,707	2,246

WHAT SHOULD YOU DRINK?

Because water is so vital to good health and helps to maximize the fat burning process, it is always your best choice when following the Formula. Refer to chapter one to determine your approximate water requirements.

Listed below are several examples of what to drink when following the Formula:

- Try to drink eight to twelve ounces of water at the start and end of each day.

- Drink six additional eight- to twelve-ounce glasses of water throughout the day, for a total of eight glasses of water or other appropriate beverages per day.

- Avoid or limit sugar and caffeinated beverages (especially beverages that contain sugar). Appropriate sugar-free and decaffeinated beverages include: water, mineral water, herbal teas, green tea, caffeine-free diet soft drinks, and decaffeinated coffee, tea, or hot water with lemon.

- If drinking fruit juice, consume only small amounts and dilute the juice with extra water.

- If you drink vegetable juice or if you use a juicer, use primarily lower glycemic vegetables such as parsley, peppers, spinach, broccoli, cabbage, and celery and reduce your consumption of the high glycemic vegetables such as carrots, beets, and apples.

- A popular 40-30-30 beverage is a lowfat decaffeinated latte, hot or iced. A latte is a coffee drink that contains steamed milk and a shot of espresso. Lowfat milk is close to the 40-30-30 ratio naturally, and with a shot of decaffeinated espresso is a delicious occasional treat for coffee lovers. You can make a mocha latte by adding unsweetened cocoa powder and a little artificial sweetener. Note: Use artificial sweeteners in moderation.

- 1% lowfat milk meets the 40-30-30 criteria naturally and can be used as part of your meal or as a snack.

- Because alcohol converts into sugar, always include a little lowfat protein with an alcoholic beverage.

Chapter Nine

FAT FLUSH BREAKFASTS

The next few chapters will provide you with recipes for delicious meals that follow the Fat Flush Formula. Before you dive right in, please read the following information about one of the ingredients called for in some of the recipes.

PURE WHEY PROTEIN POWDER

Whey protein is the newest generation of protein powder and contains an impressive amino acid profile. It is easy to digest, mixes instantly, and has no chalky aftertaste. It is basically tasteless and works extremely well when used in certain recipes.

Although there are a lot of different types of protein powders out there (made from soy, casein, or egg proteins, to name a few), we feel that whey protein is the best type to use.

When shopping for a whey protein powder, look for one that contains pure protein and nothing else. Many protein powders contain carbohydrates, fat, and artificial sweeteners and flavors.

The very best whey protein powders are 90% pure protein. To determine the percentage of purity of a protein powder, take the total serving size (in grams) and multiply by .90. The number you get should be the same as the total grams of protein listed in the nutritional information on the label. There should be one gram or less per serving of carbohydrates and fat.

The whey protein powder we use in our recipes has (per 22.2-gram scoop) 80 calories, zero grams of carbohydrates, zero grams of fat, and 20 grams of protein.

When we call for pure whey protein powder in our recipes, the measurement we use is grams. Each container of powder comes with a scoop, which equals about 20 grams of protein. Please use the following chart to aid you in measuring the grams of whey protein powder for each recipe. (For example, a quarter-scoop of powder contains 5 grams of protein.)

Pure whey protein powder can usually be found in health food stores. If you have trouble finding it, call Craig Nutraceuticals, Inc., at 800-293-1683. Ask for Pure WPI by Bioplex Nutrition.

Scoop	Grams
1/4	5
1/3	7
1/2	10
2/3	13
3/4	15
1	20

MEAL PLAN PERSONAL REQUIREMENTS

	A	B	C	D	E

KIDS' FAVORITE
Strawberry Smoothie

	A	B	C	D	E
Strawberries, fresh or frozen	1 cup	1 cup	1⅔ cups	2 cups	2⅔ cups
Water, cold	½ cup	½ cup	¾ cup	1 cup	1 cup
Pure whey protein powder	13 grams	13 grams	20 grams	30 grams	30 grams
Granulated fructose	2 tsp.	2 tsp.	1 tbsp.	1⅔ tbsp.	1½ tbsp.
Almonds, sliced	1⅓ tbsp.	1⅓ tbsp.	2⅓ tbsp.	3 tbsp.	3⅔ tbsp.

DIRECTIONS: Combine all ingredients in a blender and process until smooth. Granulated fructose can be found in health food stores.

KIDS' FAVORITE
O.J. Smoothie

	A	B	C	D	E
Orange juice	½ cup	½ cup	½ cup	1 cup	1⅓ cups
Fresh orange, peeled	½ orange	½ orange	1 orange	1 orange	1 orange
Water and/or ice cubes	½ cup	½ cup	¾ cup	¾ cup	¾ cup
Pure whey protein powder	13 grams	13 grams	20 grams	30 grams	30 grams
Almonds, sliced	1⅓ tbsp.	1⅓ tbsp.	2⅓ tbsp.	3 tbsp.	3⅔ tbsp.

DIRECTIONS: Combine all ingredients in a blender and process until smooth.

KIDS' FAVORITE
Blueberry Smoothie

	A	B	C	D	E
Blueberries, frozen	¾ cup	¾ cup	1½ cups	2 cups	2⅓ cups
Water and/or ice cubes	½ cup	½ cup	½ cup	¾ cup	¾ cup
Pure whey protein powder	13 grams	13 grams	20 grams	30 grams	30 grams
Granulated fructose	1 tsp.	1 tsp.	1 tsp.	1 tsp.	1 tbsp.
Almonds, sliced	1⅓ tbsp.	1⅓ tbsp.	2⅓ tbsp.	3 tbsp.	3⅔ tbsp.

DIRECTIONS: Combine all ingredients in a blender and process until smooth.

| MEAL PLAN PERSONAL REQUIREMENTS | | | | |
A	B	C	D	E

KIDS' FAVORITE

Peach Smoothie

	A	B	C	D	E
Peaches, fresh or frozen slices	1 cup	1 cup	1¾ cups	2½ cups	3 cups
Water and/or ice	½ cup	½ cup	½ cup	⅔ cup	⅔ cup
Pure whey protein powder	13 grams	13 grams	20 grams	30 grams	30 grams
Granulated fructose	1 tsp.	1 tsp.	1 tsp.	1 tsp.	1 tsp.
Almonds, sliced	1⅓ tbsp.	1⅓ tbsp.	2⅓ tbsp.	3 tbsp.	3⅔ tbsp.

DIRECTIONS: Combine all ingredients in a blender and process until smooth.

Cheese Omelette

	A	B	C	D	E
Eggs, whole	1	1	1	2	2
Eggs, whites only	1	1	2	3	3
Cheddar cheese, lowfat, grated	1 oz.	1 oz.	1½ oz.	1¾ oz.	2¼ oz.
Grapefruit, fresh	½	½	1	1	1¼

DIRECTIONS: Beat eggs and cook in a nonstick pan until set. Add cheese and fold over. Season with salt and pepper to taste. Serve with grapefruit.

Eggs and Bacon

	A	B	C	D	E
Eggs, whole	1	1	1	2	2
Egg, whites only	1	1	1	2	2
Canadian bacon	1 oz.	1 oz.	2 oz.	2 oz.	3 oz.
Tomato, medium, sliced	½	½	1	1	1
Grapefruit sections with juice, pink or red	⅔ cup	⅔ cup	1 cup	1⅔ cups	2 cups

DIRECTIONS: Scramble, hard-boil, or poach eggs. Serve with heated Canadian bacon, sliced tomatoes, and grapefruit sections.

MEAL PLAN PERSONAL REQUIREMENTS

KIDS' FAVORITE

Eggs and Fruit

	A	B	C	D	E
Eggs, whole	1	1	2	3	3
Eggs, whites only	2	2	3	4	5
Orange, medium	½	½	1	1½	2
Apple, medium	½	½	1	1	1

DIRECTIONS: Beat eggs and scramble in a nonstick pan until firm. Serve with sliced fruit.

Salsa Egg Scramble

	A	B	C	D	E
Eggs, whole	1	1	1	2	2
Eggs, whites only	2	2	3	4	5
Cheddar cheese, lowfat, grated	2 tsp.	2 tsp.	1 tbsp.	2 tbsp.	3 tbsp.
Salsa	2 tbsp.	2 tbsp.	3 tbsp.	4 tbsp.	4 tbsp.
Tomato, medium, sliced	⅔	⅔	1	1	2
Orange, medium	1	1	1½	2	2

DIRECTIONS: Beat eggs and scramble in a nonstick pan. Sprinkle with grated cheese and top with salsa. Serve with sliced tomatoes and fresh orange.

Cottage Cheese and Fruit Salad

	A	B	C	D	E
Cottage cheese, 2% lowfat	½ cup	½ cup	¾ cup	1 cup	1¼ cups
Nuts (almonds, pecans, or walnuts)	2 tsp.	2 tsp.	1⅓ tbsp.	2 tbsp.	2½ tbsp.
Strawberries, sliced	½ cup	½ cup	½ cup	¾ cup	1 cup
Kiwi, peeled and sliced	½	½	1	1	1
Grapes, green or red	¼ cup	¼ cup	½ cup	¾ cup	1 cup

DIRECTIONS: Top cottage cheese with nuts and serve with mixed fruit salad.

MEAL PLAN PERSONAL REQUIREMENTS

Oatmeal and Cottage Cheese

	A	B	C	D	E
Oatmeal old-fashioned, uncooked amount	⅓ cup	⅓ cup	½ cup	⅔ cup	¾ cup
Water	⅔ cup	⅔ cup	1 cup	1⅓ cups	1½ cups
Nuts (almonds, pecans, or walnuts)	2 tsp.	2 tsp.	1⅓ tbsp.	1⅔ tbsp.	2 tbsp.
Granulated fructose BR 506	½ tsp.	½ tsp.	½ tsp.	½ tsp.	½ tsp.
Milk, 1% lowfat	1 tbsp.	1 tbsp.	1 tbsp.	1 tbsp.	1 tbsp.
Cottage cheese, 2% lowfat	⅓ cup	⅓ cup	½ cup	¾ cup	1 cup

DIRECTIONS: Cook rolled oats in water per package directions. Top with chopped nuts, fructose, and milk. Serve with cottage cheese on the side or mix it into the hot cereal.

KIDS' FAVORITE
Canadian Bacon and Fruit

	A	B	C	D	E
Canadian bacon	3 oz.	3 oz.	4 oz.	5½ oz.	7 oz.
Apple, medium size	1	1	1½	2	2½

DIRECTIONS: Serve Canadian bacon cold or warmed with apple slices.

KIDS' FAVORITE
Yogurt Blend

	A	B	C	D	E
Yogurt (Knudsen Cal 70), any flavor	1	1	1	1	1
Cottage cheese, 2% lowfat	¼ cup	¼ cup	⅓ cup	⅔ cup	¾ cup
Apple, medium size	⅓	⅓	½	1	1
Nuts (almonds, pecans, or walnuts)	1⅓ tbsp.	1⅓ tbsp.	2 tbsp.	2½ tbsp.	3 tbsp.

DIRECTIONS: Combine fruit-flavored yogurt with cottage cheese and apple. Sprinkle with nuts.

	MEAL PLAN PERSONAL REQUIREMENTS				
	A	B	C	D	E

KIDS' FAVORITE

Turkey Roll-Up with Fruit

	A	B	C	D	E
Turkey, sliced deli style	1 oz.	1 oz.	2 oz.	3 oz.	4 oz.
Swiss cheese, lowfat	1 oz.	1 oz.	1½ oz.	2	2
Mustard, Dijon	1 tsp.	1 tsp.	1 tsp.	1 tsp.	1 tsp.
Mayonnaise, lowfat	1 tsp.	1 tsp.	1½ tsp.	2 tsp.	1 tbsp.
Grapes, green or red	½ cup	½ cup	½ cup	1½ cups	2 cups
Apple, medium size	½	½	1	1	1

DIRECTIONS: Place turkey on cheese with mustard and mayonnaise. Roll it up and serve with fresh fruit.

Fortified High-Fiber Cereal

	A	B	C	D	E
Bran cereal	½ cup	½ cup	⅔ cup	1 cup	1¼ cups
Pure whey protein powder	7 grams	7 grams	13 grams	15 grams	20 grams
Nuts (almonds, pecans, or walnuts)	1 tbsp.	1 tbsp.	1½ tbsp.	2½ tbsp.	3 tbsp.
Milk, 1% lowfat	⅓ cup	⅓ cup	½ cup	⅔ cup	⅔ cup

DIRECTIONS: Sprinkle bran cereal with protein powder and nuts and top with milk.

KIDS' FAVORITE

Sausage and Fruit

	A	B	C	D	E
Chicken or turkey sausage, lowfat	3 oz.	3 oz.	5 oz.	6½ oz.	7 oz.
Grapefruit sections, fresh or in a jar	1 cup	1 cup	1½ cup	2¼ cup	2½ cup

DIRECTIONS: Serve cooked sausage with grapefruit sections.

Family Style Meal

Vegetable Frittata

MEAL PLAN PERSONAL REQUIREMENTS

	A	B	C	D	E
Frittata	⅛ of pie	⅛ of pie	¼ of pie	⅜ of pie	½ of pie
Canadian bacon	1 oz.	1 oz.	1½ oz.	1½ oz.	1½ oz.
Orange sections	⅔ cup	⅔ cup	¾ cup	1¼ cups	1¼ cups

FRITTATA RECIPE

1 tablespoon olive oil

1½ cups thin-sliced onion

1 cup sliced zucchini

6 asparagus spears, sliced

¼ teaspoon salt

⅛ teaspoon pepper

3 eggs, whole

6 egg whites

¼ cup Parmesan cheese

1 tablespoon basil

1 tablespoon parsley

¼ teaspoon salt

⅛ teaspoon pepper

RECIPE DIRECTIONS: Heat oil in a large ovenproof skillet over medium heat. Add onions and cook until browned. Add zucchini and asparagus and cook about 10 more minutes. Season with salt and pepper. Turn on broiler. In a mixing bowl, beat eggs and egg whites and add cheese, herbs, and salt and pepper. Pour into hot skillet with vegetables. Cook over medium heat until the center is almost set. Place under the broiler until the top is browned, about 2 minutes. Heat Canadian bacon in a nonstick pan or microwave. Serve frittata with Canadian bacon and fruit.

MEAL PLAN PERSONAL REQUIREMENTS

	A	B	C	D	E
KIDS' FAVORITE					
40-30-30 Nutrition Bar					
40-30-30 Nutrition Bar, any flavor	1	1	1	2	2
Milk, 1% lowfat	0	0	8 oz.	8 oz.	12 oz.

DIRECTIONS: When using a 40-30-30 Nutrition Bar for a breakfast meal replacement, one bar with water, coffee, or tea is appropriate for the A or B plan. If you are following the C, D, or E plan, one bar is not enough. Have one to two bars with lowfat milk in addition to water, coffee, or tea.

	A	B	C	D	E
KIDS' FAVORITE					
40-30-30 Shake Mix					
40-30-30 Shake Mix, any flavor	1 packet	1 packet	1 packet	2 packets	2 packets
Water	8 oz.	8 oz.	4 oz.	8 oz.	8 oz.
Milk, 1% lowfat	0	0	4 oz.	8 oz.	12 oz.

DIRECTIONS: When using a 40-30-30 Shake Mix for a breakfast meal replacement, 1 packet with water is appropriate for the A or B plan. If you are following the C, D, or E plan, one packet is not enough. Have one to two packets with water and lowfat milk. For a thicker shake, use a blender and add ice cubes for part of the water.

Chapter Ten

FAT FLUSH LUNCHES

MEAL PLAN PERSONAL REQUIREMENTS

	A	B	C	D	E

KIDS' FAVORITE

Cocoa Peanut Butter Shake

	A	B	C	D	E
Milk, 1% lowfat	½ cup	¾ cup	¾ cup	1 cup	1½ cups
Cocoa powder, unsweetened	1½ tbsp.	2 tbsp.	2 tbsp.	2¼ tbsp.	2½ tbsp.
Granulated fructose	1½ tbsp.	2 tbsp.	2 tbsp.	2½ tbsp.	2⅔ tbsp.
Peanut butter, natural	1 tbsp.	1⅓ tbsp.	1⅓ tbsp.	1¾ tbsp.	2 tbsp.
Pure whey protein powder	13 grams	20 grams	20 grams	27 grams	27 grams
Ice cubes	⅔ cup	¾ cup	¾ cup	1 cup	1 cup

DIRECTIONS: Combine all ingredients in a blender and process until smooth. Natural peanut butter and granulated fructose can be found at health food stores.

KIDS' FAVORITE

Berry-Peach Smoothie

	A	B	C	D	E
Strawberries, unsweetened, fresh or frozen	⅔ cup	1 cup	1 cup	1½ cups	1½ cups
Peaches, sliced, fresh or frozen	⅔ cup	1 cup	1 cup	1 cup	1½ cups
Water	½ cup	⅔ cup	⅔ cup	¾ cup	1 cup
Pure whey protein powder	15 grams	25 grams	25 grams	30 grams	45 grams
Granulated fructose	1 tsp.	2 tsp.	2 tsp.	2 tsp.	1 tbsp.
Almonds, sliced	1¾ tbsp.	2¾ tbsp.	2¾ tbsp.	3½ tbsp.	4½ tbsp.

DIRECTIONS: Combine all ingredients in a blender and process until smooth.

	MEAL PLAN PERSONAL REQUIREMENTS				
	A	B	C	D	E

KIDS' FAVORITE

Yogurt Smoothie

	A	B	C	D	E
Plain yogurt, nonfat	1 cup	1⅓ cups	1⅓ cups	1½ cups	1¾ cups
Pure whey protein powder	7 grams	13 grams	13 grams	20 grams	25 grams
Strawberries, unsweetened, fresh or frozen	½ cup	¾ cup	¾ cup	1½ cups	2 cups
Granulated fructose	1½ tbsp.	3 tbsp.	3 tbsp.	3½ tbsp.	4½ tbsp.
Nuts (almonds, pecans, or walnuts)	1 tsp.	1½ tsp.	1½ tsp.	2 tsp.	2 tsp.

DIRECTIONS: Blend all ingredients in a blender until smooth.

Cottage Cheese and Fruit Platter

	A	B	C	D	E
Cottage cheese, 2% lowfat	½ cup	¾ cup	¾ cup	1 cup	1⅓ cups
Lettuce leaves, red leaf	3	3	3	3	3
Nuts (almonds, pecans, or walnuts)	1⅓ tbsp.	2 tbsp.	2 tbsp.	3 tbsp.	3½ tbsp.
Strawberries, sliced	½ cup	1 cup	1 cup	1 cup	1½ cups
Grapes, green or red	⅓ cup	⅔ cup	⅔ cup	¾ cup	1 cup
Apple, medium	½	½	½	1	1

DIRECTIONS: On a plate, place cottage cheese on lettuce leaves and sprinkle with nuts. Serve with sliced fruit.

Cottage Cheese Fruit Salad

	A	B	C	D	E
Cottage cheese, 2% lowfat	⅔ cup	¾ cup	¾ cup	1 cup	1⅓ cups
Strawberries, sliced	⅓ cup	⅓ cup	⅓ cup	¾ cup	1 cup
Apple, medium, sliced	½	1	1	1	1
Grapes, green or red	⅓ cup	⅓ cup	⅓ cup	¾ cup	1 cup
Nuts (almonds, pecans, or walnuts)	1⅓ tbsp.	2¼ tbsp.	2¼ tbsp.	2¾ tbsp.	3½ tbsp.
Cinnamon or nutmeg	dash	dash	dash	dash	dash

DIRECTIONS: Mix cottage cheese with sliced fruit and nuts. Sprinkle with a dash of cinnamon or nutmeg.

1-29

MEAL PLAN PERSONAL REQUIREMENTS

Tossed Tuna Salad

	A	B	C ↓	D	E
Lettuce, head, romaine or red leaf, torn	¼ head	¼ head	¼ head	½ head	½ head
Apple, medium, cored and cubed	½	1	1	1	1 large
Mandarin oranges, canned in water and drained	⅓ cup	½ cup	½ cup	¾ cup	1 cup
Albacore tuna, water packed and drained	4 oz.	6 oz.	6 oz.	8 oz.	10 oz.
Walnuts, chopped	2 tsp.	1 tbsp.	1 tbsp.	2 tbsp.	2 tbsp.
DRESSING:					
Mayonnaise, lowfat	2½ tbsp.	3 tbsp.	3 tbsp.	3 tbsp.	¼ cup
Plain yogurt, nonfat	1 tbsp.	1 tbsp.	1 tbsp.	2 tbsp.	2 tbsp.
Soy sauce	2 tsp.	2 tsp.	2 tsp.	2 tsp.	2 tsp.
Lemon juice, bottled or fresh	1 tsp.	1 tsp.	1 tsp.	2 tsp.	2 tsp.

DIRECTIONS: In a large salad bowl, combine lettuce, apple cubes, orange segments, tuna, and walnuts. In a small cup, blend mayonnaise, yogurt, soy sauce, and lemon juice. Pour over salad and toss.

KIDS' FAVORITE
Tuna Lettuce Wraps and Fruit

	A	B	C	D	E
Albacore tuna, water packed and drained	4 oz.	6 oz.	6 oz.	8 oz.	10 oz.
Celery, diced	½ stalk	½ stalk	½ stalk	1 stalk	1 stalk
Green onion, diced	1	1	1	1	1
Red cabbage, finely shredded	⅓ cup	⅔ cup	⅔ cup	1 cup	1 cup
Italian bottled salad dressing (full fat)	1½ tbsp.	2½ tbsp.	2½ tbsp.	3 tbsp.	¼ cup
Lettuce leaves, romaine or red leaf	2	4	4	6	7
Apple	1 medium	1 large	1 large	2 medium	2½ medium

DIRECTIONS: Combine tuna, celery, onion, cabbage, and Italian salad dressing. Divide tuna mixture and roll in lettuce leaves. Serve with apple slices.

MEAL PLAN PERSONAL REQUIREMENTS

	A	B	C	D	E
Tuna Stuffed Tomato					
Tomato, large	1	1	1	1	1
Albacore tuna, water packed and drained	4 oz.	6 oz.	6 oz.	8 oz.	10 oz.
Celery, diced	½ stalk	1 stalk	1 stalk	1 stalk	1 stalk
Pickle relish, sweet or dill	½ tbsp.	1 tbsp.	1 tbsp.	1 tbsp.	1 tbsp.
Onion	½ tbsp.	1 tbsp.	1 tbsp.	1 tbsp.	1 tbsp.
Black olives, large	4	4	4	7	7
Mayonnaise, lowfat	1½ tbsp.	2 tbsp.	2 tbsp.	2 tbsp.	2 tbsp.
Sunflower seeds	½ tbsp.	1 tbsp.	1 tbsp.	1½ tbsp.	1½ tbsp.
Grapes, green or red	½ cup	⅔ cup	⅔ cup	1 cup	1½ cups
Apple, medium, sliced	½	½	½	1	1

DIRECTIONS: Slice tomato horizontally and hollow out both halves. Combine tuna, celery, pickle relish, onion, black olives, and mayonnaise. Place tuna salad in tomato halves, sprinkle with sunflower seeds, and serve with fresh grapes and apple slices.

	A	B	C	D	E
Egg Salad					
Eggs, whole, hard-boiled	1	2	2	2	2
Egg whites, hard-boiled	3	4	4	6	8
Green onion, minced	1	1	1	1	2
Celery, minced	2 tbsp.	2 tbsp.	2 tbsp.	3 tbsp.	4 tbsp.
Dill pickle, whole, minced	⅓ pickle	½ pickle	½ pickle	¾ pickle	¾ pickle
Mayonnaise, lowfat	1⅓ tbsp.	1½ tbsp.	1½ tbsp.	2½ tbsp.	3½ tbsp.
Mustard, prepared	¾ tsp.	1 tsp.	1 tsp.	1¼ tsp.	1½ tsp.
Salt and pepper to taste					
Tomato, medium, sliced	1	1	1	1	2
Peach, medium	1	1	1	1	2
Bing cherries	¼ cup	⅔ cup	⅔ cup	1 cup	¾ cup

DIRECTIONS: Hard-boil eggs and cool. Peel and discard the appropriate amount of yolks. In a mixing bowl, blend chopped eggs and whites, green onions, celery, dill pickle, mayonnaise, and mustard. Add salt and pepper to taste. Serve with sliced tomatoes and fresh fruit.

MEAL PLAN PERSONAL REQUIREMENTS

	A	B	C	D	E
Chef's Salad					
Lettuce, torn	2 cups	2½ cups	2½ cups	3 cups	4 cups
Deli turkey breast, sliced	1 oz.	2 oz.	2 oz.	2½ oz.	4 oz.
Deli ham, extra lean, sliced	½ oz.	1 oz.	1 oz.	1 oz.	1 oz.
Hard-boiled egg white, diced	1	1	1	1	1
Swiss cheese, lowfat, sliced	½ oz.	½ oz.	½ oz.	1 oz.	1 oz.
Cherry tomatoes	4	4	4	6	8
Cucumber slices, peeled and seeded	¼ whole	⅓ whole	⅓ whole	⅔ whole	¾ whole
Salad dressing, reduced fat, your choice	1 tbsp.	1½ tbsp.	1½ tbsp.	2 tbsp.	2⅓ tbsp.
Pear or apple, medium	½	1	1	1	1

DIRECTIONS: Top torn lettuce with sliced turkey, ham, diced egg white, cheese, tomatoes, and cucumber and top with your favorite lowfat salad dressing. Serve with sliced pear or apple.

Joyce's Famous Chicken Caesar Salad

	A	B	C	D	E
Romaine lettuce, cleaned, dried, and torn	3 cups	3 cups	3 cups	4 cups	4 cups
Cooked chicken breast, sliced	3 oz.	3½ oz.	3½ oz.	5 oz.	6 oz.
Caesar Dressing (recipe follows)	2 tbsp.	3 tbsp.	3 tbsp.	4 tbsp.	5 tbsp.
Parmesan cheese, grated	2 tsp.	1 tbsp.	1 tbsp.	1 tbsp.	1½ tbsp.
Apple, medium	1	1	1	1	1
Grapes, green or red	0	⅔ cup	⅔ cup	1⅓ cups	2 cups

CAESAR DRESSING

1 tablespoon olive oil

1 tablespoon red wine vinegar

½ tablespoon fresh lemon juice

1 small clove of garlic, pressed, or ½ teaspoon garlic powder

½ teaspoon Worcestershire sauce

½ teaspoon anchovy paste (in tube)

½ teaspoon dry mustard powder

⅛ teaspoon pepper

⅛ teaspoon salt

CAESAR DRESSING DIRECTIONS: Place all ingredients in a small jar and shake well until blended.

OVERALL DIRECTIONS: Toss romaine lettuce and chicken with Caesar Dressing. Sprinkle with Parmesan cheese and serve salad with fruit.

MEAL PLAN PERSONAL REQUIREMENTS

Farmer's Market Salad

	A	B	C	D	E
Salad greens, any kind	2 cups	2 cups	2 cups	3 cups	3 cups
Cherry tomatoes, whole	4	5	5	6	8
Cucumber	½ cup	⅔ cup	⅔ cup	⅔ cup	1 cup
Broccoli florets	⅓ cup	¾ cup	¾ cup	¾ cup	1 cup
Snow peas	¼ cup	⅓ cup	⅓ cup	⅓ cup	½ cup
Garbanzo beans, canned, drained	¼ cup	⅓ cup	⅓ cup	½ cup	⅔ cup
Red or green bell pepper slices	¼ cup	⅓ cup	⅓ cup	⅓ cup	½ cup
Cooked chicken or albacore tuna, water packed, drained	2 oz.	3 oz.	3 oz.	4 oz.	5 oz.
Olive oil and vinegar salad dressing	1½ tbsp.	2⅓ tbsp.	2⅓ tbsp.	3 tbsp.	¼ cup

DIRECTIONS: In a large salad bowl, combine salad greens, tomatoes, cucumber, broccoli, snow peas, garbanzo beans, and peppers with chicken or tuna. Toss with salad dressing and serve.

Chinese Chicken Salad

	MEAL PLAN PERSONAL REQUIREMENTS				
	A	B	C	D	E
Cooked chicken breast, diced	2½ oz.	3½ oz.	3½ oz.	5 oz.	6 oz.
Broccoli florets	½ cup	1 cup	1 cup	1 cup	1⅓ cups
Snow peas	⅓ cup	½ cup	½ cup	¾ cup	¾ cup
Green onions, chopped	1 whole	2 whole	2 whole	3 whole	4 whole
Napa cabbage, chopped	½ cup	1 cup	1 cup	1¼ cups	1⅓ cup
Mandarin oranges, canned in natural juice, drained	½ cup	⅔ cup	⅔ cup	1 cup	1 cup
Sesame oil	½ tbsp.	1 tbsp.	1 tbsp.	1¼ tbsp.	1½ tbsp.
Rice vinegar	½ tbsp.	1 tbsp.	1 tbsp.	1¼ tbsp.	1½ tbsp.
Lemon juice	½ tbsp.	1 tbsp.	1 tbsp.	1¼ tbsp.	1½ tbsp.
Soy sauce	1 tsp.	½ tbsp.	½ tbsp.	2 tsp.	1 tbsp.
Granulated fructose	1 tsp.	½ tbsp.	½ tbsp.	2 tsp.	1 tbsp.
Ginger, ground	⅛ tsp.	⅛ tsp.	⅛ tsp.	⅛ tsp.	¼ tsp.

DIRECTIONS: Combine cooked chicken, broccoli, snow peas, green onions, cabbage, and oranges in a large bowl. In a small cup or jar, mix sesame oil, vinegar, lemon juice, soy sauce, fructose, and ginger. Pour dressing over salad and toss.

Warm Spinach and Chicken Salad

	MEAL PLAN PERSONAL REQUIREMENTS				
	A	B	C	D	E
Fresh spinach, cleaned, dried, and torn	2 cups	2½ cups	2½ cups	3 cups	4 cups
Mushrooms, whole, cleaned, dried, and sliced	3	3	3	4	4
Green onion, whole	1	1	1	2	2
Cooked chicken, cubed	2 oz.	3 oz.	3 oz.	4 oz.	5 oz.
Bacon, center cut, chopped	1 slice	2 slices	2 slices	2 slices	2 slices
Bacon fat drippings	½ tbsp.	⅔ tbsp.	⅔ tbsp.	1 tbsp.	1 tbsp.
Red wine vinegar	1 tbsp.	1½ tbsp.	1½ tbsp.	2 tbsp.	2 tbsp.
Lemon juice	1 tbsp.	1 tbsp.	1 tbsp.	1½ tbsp.	2 tbsp.
Fructose, granulated	1½ tsp.	2 tsp.	2 tsp.	1 tbsp.	1 tbsp.
Salt	⅛ tsp.	⅛ tsp.	⅛ tsp.	⅛ tsp.	⅛ tsp.
Pepper	⅛ tsp.	⅛ tsp.	⅛ tsp.	¼ tsp.	¼ tsp.
Hard-boiled egg, white only, diced	1	1	1	1	1
Apple, sliced	½ small	1 medium	1 medium	1 medium	1 large

DIRECTIONS: Place spinach in a large bowl and add sliced mushrooms, chopped onion, and cooked chicken. Just before serving, fry bacon until crisp and remove from pan. To hot bacon drippings, add vinegar, lemon juice, fructose, and salt and pepper until hot and bubbly. Pour immediately over spinach and toss. Sprinkle salad with diced egg whites and crumbled bacon. Serve with apple slices.

MEAL PLAN PERSONAL REQUIREMENTS

	D	E
oz.	5 oz.	6½ oz.
tbsp.	3 tbsp.	3 tbsp.
cup	1⅔ cups	1 cup
	1	2
tbsp.	2½ tbsp.	3 tbsp.
½ tbsp.	2 tbsp.	3 tbsp.
tsp.	1 tsp.	1 tsp.
leaves	4 leaves	4 leaves

walnuts with mayonnaise and
leaves.

	D	E
½ oz.	6 oz.	7 oz.
tbsp.	1 tbsp.	1 tbsp.
tbsp.	1 tbsp.	1 tbsp.
¼	⅓	⅓
tbsp.	2 tbsp.	3 tbsp.
tbsp.	1 tbsp.	1⅓ tbsp.
tsp.	1 tsp.	½ tbsp.
tsp.	½ tsp.	⅔ tsp.
tsp.	½ tsp.	⅔ tsp.
leaves	3 leaves	3 leaves
	1	1½
½	1	1
cup	1 cup	1⅓ cups

green onion, and avocado. In a cup, combine mayonnaise, chili sauce, lemon juice, Worcestershire sauce, and horseradish. Add to shrimp and mix well. Cut fruit into 1-inch pieces and thread on wooden picks or skewers. Serve shrimp salad on lettuce leaves with fruit kabobs.

MEAL PLAN PERSONAL REQUIREMENTS

	A	B	C	D	E
KIDS' FAVORITE					
Vegetable Chili with Fruit					
Vegetable Chili (see Vegetable Chili recipe, page 114)	1 cup	1½ cups	1½ cups	2 cups	2½ cups
Apple, medium	½	1	1	1	1

DIRECTIONS: Vegetable Chili makes great leftovers. Refer to dinner recipe and have the appropriate amount for lunch with fruit.

FAST FOOD

KIDS' FAVORITE	A	B	C	D	E
Wendy's Chili					
Wendy's chili small = 8 oz., large = 12 oz.	8 oz.	12 oz.	12 oz.	20 oz.	24 oz.

DIRECTIONS: Order appropriate amount of chili and have with water, iced tea with lemon, or a diet drink. Sorry, no Frostie or crackers!

KIDS' FAVORITE	A	B	C	D	E
Deli Meal 1					
Sliced deli meat (turkey, chicken, lean ham, or beef)	2½ oz.	3 oz.	3 oz.	4 oz.	6 oz.
Sliced Swiss cheese, 50% reduced fat	1 oz.	2 oz.	2 oz.	2½ oz.	3 oz.
Apple or pear	1 medium	1 large	1 large	1 med.+1 lg.	2 large

DIRECTIONS: In a grocery store or deli, order your specific amount of sliced deli meat and cheese and grab an apple or pear in the produce department.

KIDS' FAVORITE	A	B	C	D	E
Deli Meal 2					
Deli-prepared chicken or tuna salad	4 oz.	6 oz.	6 oz.	8 oz.	10 oz.
Apple or pear	1 medium	1 large	1 large	1 med.+1 lg.	2 large

DIRECTIONS: In a grocery store deli, order your specific amount of prepared chicken or tuna salad and grab an apple or pear in the produce department.

Chapter Eleven

FAT FLUSH SNACKS

KIDS' FAVORITE

Almond Mocha Blended Latte—Joyce's Favorite

MEAL PLAN PERSONAL REQUIREMENTS

	A	B	C	D	E
Ice cubes	1 cup	1 cup	1 cup	1 cup	2 cups
Milk, 1% lowfat	¼ cup	¼ cup	¼ cup	¼ cup	½ cup
Water	¼ cup	¼ cup	¼ cup	¼ cup	½ cup
Nescafé Decaf French Roast gourmet instant coffee	1 tsp.	1 tsp.	1 tsp.	1 tsp.	2 tsp.
Cocoa powder, unsweetened	2 tsp.	2 tsp.	2 tsp.	2 tsp.	1⅓ tbsp.
Almond butter	2 tsp.	2 tsp.	2 tsp.	2 tsp.	1⅓ tbsp.
Pure whey protein powder	15 grams	15 grams	15 grams	15 grams	30 grams
Granulated fructose	1 tbsp.	1 tbsp.	1 tbsp.	1 tbsp.	2 tbsp.

DIRECTIONS: Combine all ingredients in a blender and process until smooth. Almond butter, pure whey protein powder, and granulated fructose can be found in health food stores.

	MEAL PLAN PERSONAL REQUIREMENTS				
	A	B	C	D	E

Salad Smoothie—One of Gene's Favorites

	A	B	C	D	E
Fresh green juice (celery, spinach, cucumbers, lettuce, parsley, kale, wheat grass, greens)	8 oz.	8 oz.	8 oz.	8 oz.	16 oz.
Emer'gen-C™ packet	1	1	1	1	1
Peaches, frozen	½ cup	½ cup	½ cup	½ cup	1 cup
Pure whey protein powder	15 grams	15 grams	15 grams	15 grams	30 grams
Bee pollen	1 tsp.	1 tsp.	1 tsp.	1 tsp.	1½ tsp.
Flax oil	½ tbsp.	½ tbsp.	½ tbsp.	½ tbsp.	1 tbsp.

DIRECTIONS: Combine all ingredients in a blender and process until smooth. Juice your own greens or buy fresh bottled green juice at the health food store. Look for bottled juice without any fruit juices added. Emer'gen-C™ can be found in health food stores and is a powdered packet of vitamin C with minerals and B vitamins. Bee pollen and flax oil can be found in health food stores.

KIDS' FAVORITE
Strawberry Smoothie

	A	B	C	D	E
Strawberries, fresh or frozen	1 cup	1 cup	1 cup	1 cup	2⅔ cups
Water, cold	½ cup	½ cup	½ cup	½ cup	1 cup
Pure whey protein powder	13 grams	13 grams	13 grams	13 grams	30 grams
Granulated fructose	2 tsp.	2 tsp.	2 tsp.	2 tsp.	1½ tbsp.
Almonds, sliced	1⅓ tbsp.	1⅓ tbsp.	1⅓ tbsp.	1⅓ tbsp.	3⅔ tbsp.

DIRECTIONS: Combine all ingredients in a blender and process until smooth.

KIDS' FAVORITE
Blueberry Smoothie

	A	B	C	D	E
Blueberries, frozen	¾ cup	¾ cup	¾ cup	¾ cup	2⅓ cups
Water and/or ice	½ cup	½ cup	½ cup	½ cup	¾ cup
Pure whey protein powder	13 grams	13 grams	13 grams	13 grams	30 grams
Granulated fructose	1 tsp.	1 tsp.	1 tsp.	1 tsp.	1 tbsp.
Almonds, sliced	1⅓ tbsp.	1⅓ tbsp.	1⅓ tbsp.	1⅓ tbsp.	3⅔ tbsp.

DIRECTIONS: Combine all ingredients in a blender and process until smooth.

| | MEAL PLAN PERSONAL REQUIREMENTS | | | | |
	A	B	C	D	E

KIDS' FAVORITE

Peach Smoothie

	A	B	C	D	E
Peaches, fresh or frozen slices	1 cup	1 cup	1 cup	1 cup	3 cups
Water and/or ice	½ cup	½ cup	½ cup	½ cup	⅔ cup
Pure whey protein powder	13 grams	13 grams	13 grams	13 grams	30 grams
Granulated fructose	1 tsp.	1 tsp.	1 tsp.	1 tsp.	1 tsp.
Almonds, sliced	1⅓ tbsp.	1⅓ tbsp.	1⅓ tbsp.	1⅓ tbsp.	3⅔ tbsp.

DIRECTIONS: Combine all ingredients in a blender and process until smooth.

KIDS' FAVORITE

40-30-30 Nutrition Bar

	A	B	C	D	E
40-30-30 Nutrition Bar, any flavor	1	1	1	1	2

DIRECTIONS: Have a 40-30-30 Nutrition Bar with water, decaffeinated coffee, or tea.

KIDS' FAVORITE

40-30-30 Shake Mix

	A	B	C	D	E
40-30-30 Shake Mix, any flavor	1 packet	1 packet	1 packet	1 packet	2 packets
Water	8 oz.	8 oz.	8 oz.	8 oz.	16 oz.

DIRECTIONS: Blend 40-30-30 shake mix with water. For a thicker shake, use a blender and add ice cubes for part of the water.

Knudsen Cottage Doubles

	A	B	C	D	E
Knudsen Cottage Doubles (single-serving size)	1	1	1	1	2
Nuts (almonds, pecans, or walnuts)	2 tsp.	2 tsp.	2 tsp.	2 tsp.	1⅓ tbsp.

DIRECTIONS: Have Knudsen Cottage Doubles with added nuts.

MEAL PLAN PERSONAL REQUIREMENTS

	A	B	C	D	E
Lowfat Cottage Cheese with Fruit					
Knudsen on the Go! Lowfat 2%					
Milkfat Cottage Cheese (4-oz. cup)	1	1	1	1	2
Nuts (almonds, pecans, or walnuts)	2 tsp.	2 tsp.	2 tsp.	2 tsp.	1⅓ tbsp.
Apple, medium size	½	½	½	½	1

DIRECTIONS: Have cottage cheese with added nuts and sliced apple.

	A	B	C	D	E
Lowfat Cottage Cheese and Fruit					
Knudsen on the Go! Lowfat Cottage					
Cheese & Fruit (4-oz. cup)	1	1	1	1	2
Nuts (almonds, pecans, or walnuts)	1 tsp.	1 tsp.	1 tsp.	1 tsp.	2 tsp.

DIRECTIONS: Have cottage cheese and fruit with added nuts.

	A	B	C	D	E
Soybeans and Grapes					
Soybeans, raw	¼ cup	¼ cup	¼ cup	¼ cup	½ cup
Grapes or bing cherries	8	8	8	8	16

DIRECTIONS: Eat soybeans with grapes or cherries.

KIDS' FAVORITE

	A	B	C	D	E
Deli Tuna Salad on Apple Slices					
Tuna salad (prepared with lowfat					
mayonnaise)	3 oz.	3 oz.	3 oz.	3 oz.	6 oz.
Apple, medium	1	1	1	1	2

DIRECTIONS: Place deli-style tuna salad on apple slices.

MEAL PLAN PERSONAL REQUIREMENTS

	A	B	C	D	E

KIDS' FAVORITE

Deli Meat Roll-Up

	A	B	C	D	E
Deli meat, sliced (chicken, turkey, ham, or beef)	1 oz.	1 oz.	1 oz.	1 oz.	2 oz.
Swiss cheese, lowfat, sliced	1 oz.	1 oz.	1 oz.	1 oz.	2 oz.
Small apple or pear	1	1	1	1	2

DIRECTIONS: Place deli meat on cheese and roll up. Serve with fruit.

Deli Meat Slices and Coleslaw

	A	B	C	D	E
Deli meat, sliced (chicken or turkey)	3 oz.	3 oz.	3 oz.	3 oz.	6 oz.
Deli-made coleslaw	4 oz.	4 oz.	4 oz.	4 oz.	8 oz.

DIRECTIONS: Have deli-sliced chicken or turkey with coleslaw.

KIDS' FAVORITE

Peanut Butter Yogurt

	A	B	C	D	E
Yogurt, plain, nonfat (Dannon)	8 oz.	8 oz.	8 oz.	8 oz.	16 oz.
Peanut butter, natural	1 tbsp.	1 tbsp.	1 tbsp.	1 tbsp.	2 tbsp.
Granulated fructose	2 tsp.	2 tsp.	2 tsp.	2 tsp.	1⅓ tbsp.
Pure whey protein powder	5 grams	5 grams	5 grams	5 grams	10 grams

DIRECTIONS: Stir peanut butter, fructose, and pure whey protein powder into plain yogurt.

KIDS' FAVORITE

Fruit with Yogurt Dip

	A	B	C	D	E
Yogurt, plain, nonfat (Dannon)	⅓ cup	⅓ cup	⅓ cup	⅓ cup	⅔ cup
Pure whey protein powder	10 grams	10 grams	10 grams	10 grams	30 grams
Granulated fructose	1 tsp.	1 tsp.	1 tsp.	1 tsp.	2 tsp.
Walnuts, diced	1 tbsp.	1 tbsp.	1 tbsp.	1 tbsp.	2 tbsp.
Apple, medium, thinly sliced	½	½	½	½	1

DIRECTIONS: Combine yogurt with pure whey protein powder, fructose, and walnuts. Use as a dip for apples.

MEAL PLAN PERSONAL REQUIREMENTS

	A	B	C	D	E

KIDS' FAVORITE

Nutty Sweet Yogurt

	A	B	C	D	E
Yogurt, plain, nonfat (Dannon)	8 oz.	8 oz.	8 oz.	8 oz.	16 oz.
Pure whey protein powder	5 grams	5 grams	5 grams	5 grams	10 grams
Granulated fructose	1 tsp.	1 tsp.	1 tsp.	1 tsp.	2 tsp.
Nuts (almonds, pecans, or walnuts), sliced	1¾ tbsp.	1¾ tbsp.	1¾ tbsp.	1¾ tbsp.	3½ tbsp.

DIRECTIONS: Combine yogurt with pure whey protein powder, fructose, and nuts.

Fresh Fruit and Cottage Cheese

	A	B	C	D	E
Cottage cheese, 2% lowfat	½ cup	½ cup	½ cup	½ cup	1 cup
Nuts (almonds, pecans, or walnuts), chopped	1 tbsp.	1 tbsp.	1 tbsp.	1 tbsp.	2 tbsp.
Choose one fruit:					
Cherries (⅔ cup = about 15)	⅔ cup	⅔ cup	⅔ cup	⅔ cup	1⅓ cups
Grapes (½ cup = about 20)	½ cup	½ cup	½ cup	½ cup	1 cup
Peach slices (¾ cup = 1½ peaches)	¾ cup	¾ cup	¾ cup	¾ cup	1½ cups
Strawberries	1½ cups	1½ cups	1½ cups	1½ cups	3 cups
Pear (⅔ cup = about 1 pear)	⅔ cup	⅔ cup	⅔ cup	⅔ cup	1⅓ cups
Plum (¾ cup = about 2 plums)	¾ cup	¾ cup	¾ cup	¾ cup	1½ cups
Apple (1 cup = about ⅔ apple)	1 cup	1 cup	1 cup	1 cup	2 cups
Apricot (1 cup = about 6 apricots)	1 cup	1 cup	1 cup	1 cup	2 cups
Pineapple	¾ cup	¾ cup	¾ cup	¾ cup	1½ cups

DIRECTIONS: Sprinkle nuts on top of cottage cheese and serve with your choice of fruit.

MEAL PLAN PERSONAL REQUIREMENTS				
A	B	C	D	E

Veggies with Blue Cheese Dip

	A	B	C	D	E
Cottage cheese, 2% lowfat	⅓ cup	⅓ cup	⅓ cup	⅓ cup	⅔ cup
Crumbled blue cheese	2 tbsp.	2 tbsp.	2 tbsp.	2 tbsp.	4 tbsp.
Sour cream, nonfat	2 tbsp.	2 tbsp.	2 tbsp.	2 tbsp.	4 tbsp.
Worcestershire sauce	¼ tsp.	¼ tsp.	¼ tsp.	¼ tsp.	½ tsp.
Vinegar	dash	dash	dash	dash	dash
Garlic powder	dash	dash	dash	dash	dash
Celery stalks, sliced	2	2	2	2	4
Cucumber, medium, seeded and sliced	½	½	½	½	1
Red or green bell peppers, medium, sliced	½	½	½	½	1

DIRECTIONS: Combine cottage cheese, blue cheese, and sour cream with a blender or food processor. Season with Worcestershire sauce, vinegar, and garlic powder. Serve as dip with sliced vegetables.

KIDS' FAVORITE

Fruit and Cheese Kabobs

	A	B	C	D	E
Apple or pear, medium size, cored and cut into chunks	½	½	½	½	1
Grapes, green or red	10	10	10	10	20
Cheese, 50% reduced fat, cut into cubes	2 oz.	2 oz.	2 oz.	2 oz.	4 oz.

DIRECTIONS: Thread apple or pear chunks, grapes, and cheese on wooden skewers.

Brands of cheese to look for: Mini Babybel Light, Laughing Cow, Sargento Moo Town Snackers Light, Land O Lakes 50% Reduced Fat, Alpine Lace Reduced Fat, Heluva Good Reduced Fat, Kraft Reduced Fat.

| | MEAL PLAN PERSONAL REQUIREMENTS | | | | |
	A	B	C	D	E

String Cheese and Grapes

	A	B	C	D	E
String cheese, lowfat	2 oz.	2 oz.	2 oz.	2 oz.	4 oz.
Grapes, green or red	¾ cup	¾ cup	¾ cup	¾ cup	1½ cups

DIRECTIONS: Have string cheese with grapes.

Hard-Boiled Eggs and Apple

	A	B	C	D	E
Egg, whole	1	1	1	1	2
Egg whites	2	2	2	2	4
Apple, medium, sliced	1	1	1	1	2

DIRECTIONS: Hard-boil eggs. Peel cooled eggs and discard the appropriate amount of yolks. Add salt and pepper to taste and serve with apple slices.

Chicken Salad in Celery Stalks

	A	B	C	D	E
Chicken breast, cooked and diced	1½ oz.	1½ oz.	1½ oz.	1½ oz.	3 oz.
Apple, medium, diced	½	½	½	½	1
Black olives, chopped	3	3	3	3	6
Mayonnaise, lowfat	1½ tbsp.	1½ tbsp.	1½ tbsp.	1½ tbsp.	3 tbsp.
Celery stalks	2	2	2	2	4

DIRECTIONS: Combine cooked chicken, apple, olives, and mayonnaise. Serve in celery stalks.

Chicken Fruit Skewers

	A	B	C	D	E
Chicken breast, cooked, cooled, and cubed	2 oz.	2 oz.	2 oz.	2 oz.	4 oz.
Black olives, large	3	3	3	3	6
Grapes, red	10	10	10	10	20
Apple, medium size, cored and cubed	½	½	½	½	1

DIRECTIONS: Alternate chicken, olives, grapes, and apple chunks on wooden skewers.

	MEAL PLAN PERSONAL REQUIREMENTS				
	A	**B**	**C**	**D**	**E**
Wine and Cheese					
Red or white wine	4 oz.	4 oz.	4 oz.	4 oz.	8 oz.
Cheese, 50% reduced fat	2 oz.	2 oz.	2 oz.	2 oz.	4 oz.

DIRECTIONS: Have wine with cheese.

KIDS' FAVORITE

Peanut Butter Spread on Apples					
Peanut butter, natural	1 tbsp.	1 tbsp.	1 tbsp.	1 tbsp.	2 tbsp.
Pure whey protein powder	13 grams	13 grams	13 grams	13 grams	26 grams
Milk, 1% lowfat	1 tbsp.	1 tbsp.	1 tbsp.	1 tbsp.	2 tbsp.
Granulated fructose	1 tsp.	1 tsp.	1 tsp.	1 tsp.	2 tsp.
Apple, small size, cored and sliced thin	1	1	1	1	2

DIRECTIONS: In a small bowl, mix together peanut butter, pure whey protein powder, milk, and fructose until smooth. Serve on thin apple slices.

Hummus Dip and Vegetables					
Garbanzo beans, canned, drained, and rinsed	½ cup	½ cup	½ cup	½ cup	1 cup
Plain yogurt, nonfat	2 tbsp.	2 tbsp.	2 tbsp.	2 tbsp.	⅓ cup
Lemon juice	½ tbsp.	½ tbsp.	½ tbsp.	½ tbsp.	1 tbsp.
Garlic clove, pressed	1	1	1	1	2
Dried pepper flakes	¼ tsp.	¼ tsp.	¼ tsp.	¼ tsp.	½ tsp.
Pure whey protein powder	10 grams	10 grams	10 grams	10 grams	20 grams
Celery stalks	2	2	2	2	4
Green or red bell peppers, medium	1	1	1	1	3

DIRECTIONS: In a small food processor, blend garbanzo beans, yogurt, lemon juice, garlic, pepper flakes, and pure whey protein powder until almost smooth. Remove bowl and store covered in refrigerator for at least 4 hours or overnight to blend flavors. Serve with sliced celery and red or green bell pepper slices.

Chapter Twelve

FAT FLUSH DINNERS

	MEAL PLAN PERSONAL REQUIREMENTS				
	A	B	C	D	E

KIDS' FAVORITE

Cocoa Peanut Butter Shake

	A	B	C	D	E
Milk, 1% lowfat	¾ cup	¾ cup	1 cup	1 cup	1¼ cups
Cocoa powder, unsweetened	2 tbsp.	2 tbsp.	2¼ tbsp.	2¼ tbsp.	2⅓ tbsp.
Granulated fructose	2 tbsp.	2⅓ tbsp.	2½ tbsp.	2½ tbsp.	3 tbsp.
Peanut butter, natural	1⅓ tbsp.	1½ tbsp.	1¾ tbsp.	1¾ tbsp.	2¼ tbsp.
Pure whey protein powder	20 grams	23 grams	27 grams	27 grams	30 grams
Ice cubes	1 cup	1 cup	1 cup	1 cup	1 cup

DIRECTIONS: Combine all ingredients in a blender and process until smooth.

KIDS' FAVORITE

Strawberry Smoothie

	A	B	C	D	E
Strawberries, fresh or frozen	2 cups	2 cups	2⅔ cups	2⅔ cups	3 cups
Water, cold	1 cup	1 cup	1 cup	1 cup	1¼ cups
Pure whey protein powder	25 grams	27 grams	33 grams	33 grams	40 grams
Granulated fructose	1⅓ tbsp.	1⅔ tbsp.	1½ tbsp.	1½ tbsp.	2 tbsp.
Almonds, sliced	2¾ tbsp.	3 tbsp.	3⅔ tbsp.	3⅔ tbsp.	¼ cup + 1 tsp.

DIRECTIONS: Combine all ingredients in a blender and process until smooth.

	MEAL PLAN PERSONAL REQUIREMENTS				
	A	B	C	D	E

KIDS' FAVORITE

Chicken and Vegetable Kabobs

	A	B	C	D	E
Chicken or turkey breast, cubed (weight before cooking)	4 oz.	5 oz.	6 oz.	6 oz.	7½ oz.
Teriyaki marinade, bottled (Kikkoman, Chung King, etc.)	2 tbsp.	3 tbsp.	3 tbsp.	3 tbsp.	3 tbsp.
Sweet onion, cut in 1-inch pieces	½ cup	½ cup	½ cup	½ cup	¾ cup
Cherry tomatoes, whole	6	8	8	8	8
Green or red bell pepper, medium	½	½	¾	¾	¾
Zucchini (about 5 to 6 inches long), cubed	1	1	1	1	1
Applesauce, unsweetened	¼ cup	½ cup	⅔ cup	⅔ cup	1 cup
Mixed salad greens	2 cups	2 cups	2½ cups	2½ cups	3 cups
Salad dressing, bottled, full-fat	1½ tbsp.	1½ tbsp.	2 tbsp.	2 tbsp.	2⅓ tbsp.

DIRECTIONS: Using bottled teriyaki sauce, marinate chicken cubes for 15 to 30 minutes. Cut vegetables into bite-size pieces. Alternate chicken and pieces of onion, whole cherry tomatoes, pepper, and zucchini on metal or bamboo skewers. Broil or grill over hot coals until done. Make sure that chicken is cooked through until white, not pink or red. Do not overcook. Serve with applesauce and a mixed green salad with your choice of dressing.

Marinated Beef Kabobs

MARINADE

1 tablespoon olive oil
1 tablespoon red wine vinegar
2 teaspoons Dijon mustard
1 teaspoon lemon juice
1 clove garlic, pressed
1 teaspoon salt

	MEAL PLAN PERSONAL REQUIREMENTS				
	A	B	C	D	E
½ teaspoon pepper					
Beef tenderloin, trimmed of fat (weight before cooking)	3 oz.	4 oz.	5 oz.	5 oz.	6½ oz.
Green or red bell pepper, medium size, cubed	⅓	⅓	½	½	½
Sweet onion, large, cubed	⅓	⅓	½	½	½
Cherry tomatoes, whole	6	6	8	8	10
Zucchini (about 5–6″ long), cubed	1	1	1	1	1
Snow peas	½ cup	½ cup	½ cup	½ cup	½ cup
Mushrooms, small	⅓ cup	⅓ cup	½ cup	½ cup	½ cup
Barley, cooked amount (see package directions)	⅓ cup	½ cup	½ cup	½ cup	¾ cup

DIRECTIONS: Blend marinade ingredients in a small cup and pour over cubed beef. Cover and refrigerate at least 15 minutes or more. Thread marinated meat and vegetables onto metal skewers or water-soaked bamboo skewers. Broil or grill over hot coals 8 to 10 minutes, turning occasionally. Serve at once over cooked barley.

	MEAL PLAN PERSONAL REQUIREMENTS				
	A	B	C	D	E

Shrimp Kabobs with Fried Barley

	A	B	C	D	E
Shrimp, large (peel all but tail)	4 oz.	4½ oz.	6 oz.	6 oz.	7½ oz.

FRIED BARLEY

	A	B	C	D	E
Pearl barley, cooked	⅔ cup	¾ cup	1 cup	1 cup	1¼ cups
Olive oil	½ tbsp.	2 tsp.	2 tsp.	2 tsp.	2 tsp.
Celery, diced	3 tbsp.	¼ cup	¼ cup	¼ cup	¼ cup
Red or white onion, diced	3 tbsp.	¼ cup	¼ cup	¼ cup	¼ cup
Broccoli, diced	3 tbsp.	¼ cup	¼ cup	¼ cup	¼ cup
Soy sauce	½ tbsp.	½ tbsp.	½ tbsp.	½ tbsp.	½ tbsp.
Eggs, whites only	2	2	2	2	2
Mixed salad greens	2 cups	2 cups	2 cups	2 cups	2 cups
Oil and vinegar dressing, bottled	2 tsp.	2 tsp.	1 tbsp.	1 tbsp.	1⅓ tbsp.

FRIED BARLEY DIRECTIONS: In a large nonstick skillet or wok, heat olive oil and lightly brown celery, onion, and broccoli just until tender. Move to the side and add egg whites and cook until set. Mix in cooked barley, vegetables, and soy sauce.

DIRECTIONS: Clean and peel shrimp, leaving tails. Thread shrimp on a metal or water-soaked bamboo skewer all facing the same direction. Brush with lemon juice and a sprinkle of garlic salt before and while grilling. Serve grilled shrimp with fried barley and a mixed green salad with dressing.

	MEAL PLAN PERSONAL REQUIREMENTS				
	A	B	C	D	E

KIDS' FAVORITE/ *Family Style*

Orange Chicken Stir-Fry

	A	B	C	D	E
Orange Chicken Stir-Fry (recipe below)	1¼ cups	1⅓ cups	1½ cups	1½ cups	2 cups
Pearl barley, cooked	½ cup	⅔ cup	¾ cup	¾ cup	1 cup

ORANGE CHICKEN STIR-FRY

1½ pounds chicken breast, cubed

8 green onions, cut into 2-inch pieces

2 tablespoons soy sauce

2 tablespoons dry cooking sherry

½ teaspoon ground ginger

½ teaspoon red pepper flakes

1½ tablespoons cornstarch

1 teaspoon granulated fructose

1 teaspoon salt

1 cup orange juice

2 large oranges, peeled and sectioned

1½ tablespoons peanut oil

½ cup walnut pieces

ORANGE CHICKEN DIRECTIONS: Cut chicken breasts into 1-inch cubes. In a bowl, mix chicken, green onions, soy sauce, sherry, ginger, and pepper flakes. Cover, and refrigerate 20 minutes or longer. In a small cup, blend cornstarch, fructose, salt, and orange juice. Heat peanut oil in skillet or wok over high heat. Add chicken mixture and stir-fry until lightly browned. Stir juice mixture and add to chicken; heat until the sauce boils and thickens. Gently mix in orange segments and walnuts.

DIRECTIONS: Serve Orange Chicken Stir-Fry over hot cooked barley.

MEAL PLAN PERSONAL REQUIREMENTS

	A	B	C	D	E

Family Style

Beef Stir-Fry with Barley

	A	B	C	D	E
Beef Stir-Fry (recipe below)	1½ cups	1⅔ cups	1¾ cups	1¾ cups	2 cups
Pearl barley, cooked	⅔ cup	⅔ cup	⅞ cup	⅞ cup	1⅛ cups

BEEF STIR-FRY

1½ pounds beef tenderloin

3 tablespoons soy sauce

3 tablespoons dry cooking sherry

1 clove garlic, pressed

1 teaspoon ground ginger

1 teaspoon red pepper flakes

4 cups chopped broccoli

4 cups sliced asparagus (2-inch slices)

2 cups mushroom pieces

1½ tablespoons cornstarch

1 cup beef broth, canned

2 tablespoons peanut oil, divided

BEEF STIR-FRY DIRECTIONS: Trim beef of visible fat and cut into ½-inch-wide by 2-inch-long strips. In a bowl, mix beef strips, soy sauce, sherry, garlic, ginger, and pepper flakes. Cover and refrigerate for at least 20 minutes. Heat 1 tablespoon of the peanut oil in a skillet or wok over high heat. Stir-fry beef mixture until browned; remove from pan. Add remaining tablespoon peanut oil to wok and stir-fry the broccoli and asparagus for about 3 minutes or until vegetables are tender-crisp. Add mushrooms for about 1 minute more. Whisk cornstarch and beef broth in a small bowl and add to vegetables, stirring until sauce boils and thickens.

DIRECTIONS: Serve Beef Stir-Fry over hot cooked barley.

	MEAL PLAN PERSONAL REQUIREMENTS				
	A	B	C	D	E

Family Style

Sweet and Sour Shrimp Stir-Fry

	A	B	C	D	E
Sweet and Sour Shrimp Stir-Fry (recipe below)	1 cup	1⅓ cups	1¾ cups	1¾ cups	2 cups
Pearl barley, cooked	½ cup	½ cup	⅔ cup	⅔ cup	¾ cup
Macadamia nuts, chopped	1¼ tbsp.	1¼ tbsp.	1½ tbsp.	1½ tbsp.	2 tbsp.

SWEET AND SOUR SHRIMP

2 tablespoons cornstarch

2 tablespoons granulated fructose

¼ teaspoon ground ginger

2 tablespoons soy sauce

2 tablespoons dry cooking sherry

¼ cup white vinegar

¼ cup chicken broth

2 tablespoons peanut oil

2 cups chopped onion

2 cups chopped green bell pepper

2 pounds medium shrimp, shelled

2 cups drained pineapple chunks

SWEET AND SOUR SHRIMP DIRECTIONS: In a small cup, blend cornstarch, fructose, ginger, soy sauce, sherry, vinegar, and broth. In a large skillet or wok, heat peanut oil and add onion and green pepper. Stir-fry until just tender and beginning to brown. Add shrimp and stir-fry until no longer translucent. Stir the sweet and sour mixture and add to vegetables and shrimp. Stir until bubbly and thick. Add pineapple chunks.

DIRECTIONS: Serve Sweet and Sour Shrimp over hot cooked barley and sprinkle with chopped macadamia nuts.

MEAL PLAN PERSONAL REQUIREMENTS

	A	B	C	D	E
Cottage Cheese and Fruit Platter					
Lettuce leaves, red leaf or romaine	2	3	3	3	3
Cottage Cheese, 2% lowfat	⅞ cup	1 cup	1¼ cups	1¼ cups	1½ cups
Nuts (almonds, pecans, or walnuts)	1 tsp.	1 tsp.	2 tsp.	2 tsp.	2 tsp.
Strawberries	½ cup	⅔ cup	1 cup	1 cup	1 cup
Grapes, green or red	½ cup	½ cup	⅔ cup	⅔ cup	1 cup
Apple, medium, sliced	½	½	½	½	½
Avocado, medium	¼	¼	¼	¼	⅓

DIRECTIONS: Place lettuce leaves on a dinner plate and top with cottage cheese. Sprinkle with sliced nuts. Surround with fresh fruit and avocado slices.

Citrus Spinach Salad

	A	B	C	D	E
Cooked chicken breast, cubed	3½ oz.	4 oz.	5 oz.	5 oz.	6 oz.
Baby spinach leaves, washed and dried	2½ cups	2½ cups	3 cups	3 cups	4 cups
Grapefruit, sections only	¾ cup	¾ cup	1 cup	1 cup	1¼ cups
Navel orange, peeled and sectioned	½ cup	¾ cup	¾ cup	¾ cup	1 cup
Avocado, medium, peeled and diced	3 tbsp.	3 tbsp.	¼ cup	¼ cup	⅓ cup

TANGERINE SHALLOT DRESSING

1 clove garlic, peeled

¼ teaspoon salt

2 tablespoons tangerine juice

2 tablespoons fresh lemon juice

1 tablespoon minced shallots

½ tablespoon olive oil

TANGERINE SHALLOT DRESSING DIRECTIONS: Mash garlic with salt to make a paste. Place in a small jar and add tangerine and lemon juices, shallots, and olive oil and shake well. (Dressing recipe can be doubled or more, then split evenly if you make more than one portion of salad.)

DIRECTIONS: In a large bowl combine chicken, spinach leaves, grapefruit, and orange. Toss with Tangerine Shallot Dressing and serve topped with diced avocado.

	MEAL PLAN PERSONAL REQUIREMENTS				
	A	B	C	D	E

Mediterranean Salad with Chicken

	A	B	C	D	E
Cooked chicken breast, diced	3 oz.	3½ oz.	4 oz.	4 oz.	5 oz.
Cucumber slices	⅓ cup	⅓ cup	½ cup	½ cup	½ cup
Red and/or green bell peppers, sliced	½ cup	½ cup	½ cup	½ cup	½ cup
Fresh tomato chunks	½ cup	½ cup	⅔ cup	⅔ cup	1 cup
Red onion, sliced	¼ cup	¼ cup	¼ cup	¼ cup	¼ cup
Kalamata olives	3	3	4	4	5
Garbanzo beans, canned, drained	⅓ cup	½ cup	½ cup	½ cup	¾ cup
Feta cheese, reduced fat, crumbled	⅓ oz.	½ oz.	½ oz.	½ oz.	¾ oz.
Romaine lettuce leaves, cleaned, dried, and torn	1½ cups	1½ cups	2 cups	2 cups	2 cups
Lemon juice	1½ tbsp.	1½ tbsp.	1½ tbsp.	1½ tbsp.	1½ tbsp.
Red wine vinegar	1½ tbsp.	1½ tbsp.	1½ tbsp.	1½ tbsp.	1½ tbsp.
Olive oil	½ tbsp.	½ tbsp.	2 tsp.	2 tsp.	2 tsp.
Dried oregano	1 tsp.	1 tsp.	1 tsp.	1 tsp.	1 tsp.
Garlic, minced	1 tsp.	1 tsp.	1 tsp.	1 tsp.	1 tsp.
Salt and pepper					

DIRECTIONS: In a large bowl, combine chicken, cucumbers, red and green peppers, tomatoes, onion, olives, garbanzo beans, feta cheese, and lettuce. In a small measuring cup, whisk lemon juice, vinegar, olive oil, oregano, garlic, and salt and pepper to taste. Pour over salad and toss well.

MEAL PLAN PERSONAL REQUIREMENTS

Cherry Chicken Salad

	A	B	C	D	E
Cooked chicken or turkey breast, diced	3 oz.	3½ oz.	4 oz.	4 oz.	5 oz.
Dried cherries	¼ cup	⅓ cup	⅓ cup	⅓ cup	⅓ cup
Walnuts, chopped	1⅓ tbsp.	1½ tbsp.	2 tbsp.	2 tbsp.	2 tbsp.
Romaine lettuce leaves	2 leaves	2 leaves	2 leaves	2 leaves	2 leaves
Cream Cheese Dressing (recipe below)	2 tbsp.	2 tbsp.	2½ tbsp.	2½ tbsp.	3 tbsp.
Three Bean Salad (recipe below)	½ cup	½ cup	¾ cup	¾ cup	1¼ cups

CREAM CHEESE DRESSING

2 ounces ⅓-less-fat cream cheese

⅛ teaspoon paprika

1 teaspoon canola oil

1 tablespoon orange juice

1 tablespoon lemon juice

¼ teaspoon salt

⅛ teaspoon pepper

CREAM CHEESE DRESSING DIRECTIONS: Combine all ingredients in a small food processor and blend until smooth and creamy.

THREE BEAN SALAD

1 cup canned green beans, drained and rinsed

¾ cup canned kidney beans, drained and rinsed

¾ cup canned garbanzo beans, drained and rinsed

¼ cup diced onion

¼ cup sliced red and green bell peppers

3 tablespoons red wine vinegar

1 tablespoon olive oil
2 teaspoons granulated fructose
1 clove garlic, pressed
½ teaspoon oregano

THREE BEAN SALAD DIRECTIONS: In a large bowl, add beans, onion, and bell pepper. In a small mixing cup, blend vinegar, oil, fructose, garlic, and oregano. Pour over bean mixture and mix well. Cover and refrigerate.

DIRECTIONS: Combine diced chicken, cherries, and walnuts. Blend in Cream Cheese Dressing. Serve chicken salad on romaine lettuce leaves with Three Bean Salad.

MEAL PLAN PERSONAL REQUIREMENTS

Chicken Caesar Salad

	A	B	C	D	E
Romaine lettuce, washed, dried, and torn	⅓ head	⅓ head	½ head	½ head	½ head
Cooked chicken breast, sliced	4½ oz.	5½ oz.	6 oz.	6 oz.	7 oz.
Caesar Dressing (recipe below)	2¼ tbsp.	2½ tbsp.	3 tbsp.	3 tbsp.	3 tbsp.
Parmesan cheese, grated	1 tbsp.	1 tbsp.	1½ tbsp.	1½ tbsp.	2½ tbsp.
Apple, medium, sliced	½	1	1	1	1
Grapes, green or red	¾ cup	⅔ cup	¾ cup	¾ cup	1¼ cups

CAESAR DRESSING

2 tablespoons olive oil
2 tablespoons red wine vinegar
1 tablespoon fresh lemon juice
1 clove of garlic, pressed, or
   1 teaspoon garlic powder
1 teaspoon Worcestershire sauce
1 teaspoon anchovy paste (in tube)

1 teasp
¼ teas
¼ tea

CAES   shake well until
blen

DIF   . Sprinkle with
Pa

	REQUIREMENTS		
	D	E	
	½ oz.	6½ oz.	8 oz.
	2 cups	2 cups	3 cups
	1¾ tbsp.	1¾ tbsp.	2⅓ tbsp.
	2 cups	2 cups	2 cups
	1½ cups	1½ cups	2 cups

¼ cup orange j
2 teaspoons Worcestershire sa
1 teaspoon salt
¼ teaspoon pepper
½ teaspoon dry mustard
1 teaspoon olive oil

LEMON MARINADE DIRECTIONS: In a small cup, whisk together all ingredients.

DIRECTIONS: Pour Lemon Marinade over chicken breast. Cover and refrigerate for at least 1 hour. Meanwhile, combine grated cabbage with oil and vinegar dressing, cover, and refrigerate. Grill or broil chicken until cooked through. Serve with cooked green beans, cabbage salad, and peaches.

MEAL PLAN PERSONAL REQUIREMENTS

Grilled Beef Dinner

	A	B	C	D	E
Extra-lean beef	4 oz.	4½ oz.	5½ oz.	5½ oz.	7 oz.
Mushrooms	1 cup	1 cup	1 cup	1 cup	1⅓ cups
Butter	½ tbsp.	½ tbsp.	½ tbsp.	½ tbsp.	2 tsp.
Tomato, medium, sliced	1	1	1	1	1
Applesauce, unsweetened	¾ cup	1¼ cups	1⅓ cups	1⅓ cups	1¾ cups
Asparagus spears, steamed	10	10	10	10	12

DIRECTIONS: Grill steak. In a small pan, sauté mushrooms in butter. Serve steak with mushrooms, sliced tomatoes, applesauce, and steamed asparagus.

KIDS' FAVORITE
Grilled Burger Patty Dinner

	A	B	C	D	E
Extra-lean ground sirloin	4 oz.	4½ oz.	5½ oz.	5½ oz.	6½ oz.
Green beans, fresh, or canned and drained	1 cup	1½ cups	2 cups	2 cups	2 cups
Sliced tomato, medium	1	1	1	1	1
Olive oil	1½ tsp.	2 tsp.	2 tsp.	2 tsp.	2½ tsp.
Green onion, diced	¼ cup	⅓ cup	⅓ cup	⅓ cup	½ cup
Mushroom pieces	¼ cup	⅓ cup	⅓ cup	⅓ cup	½ cup
Pearl barley, cooked	½ cup	½ cup	⅔ cup	⅔ cup	¾ cup
Soy sauce	½ tsp.	½ tsp.	½ tsp.	½ tsp.	1 tsp.

DIRECTIONS: Grill burger patty and season with salt, pepper, and garlic to taste. Meanwhile, heat oil in a small skillet, and sauté green onion and mushroom pieces until brown. Add cooked barley and soy sauce. Serve with green beans and sliced tomatoes.

MEAL PLAN PERSONAL REQUIREMENTS

KIDS' FAVORITE

Pork Chops and Applesauce

	A	B	C	D	E
Pork loin butterfly chop	4 oz.	4½ oz.	5 oz.	5 oz.	6½ oz.
Applesauce, unsweetened	1 cup	1¼ cups	1⅓ cups	1⅓ cups	1¾ cups
Broccoli florets, cooked	1¾ cups	2 cups	2 cups	2 cups	2 cups
Mixed salad greens	2 cups	2 cups	2 cups	2 cups	3 cups
Oil and vinegar salad dressing	1 tbsp.	1 tbsp.	1½ tbsp.	1½ tbsp.	1½ tbsp.

DIRECTIONS: Preheat oven to 375°F. Salt and pepper both sides of pork chop and add a dash of soy sauce. Heat a nonstick pan and quickly brown both sides of pork chop. Cover and place in oven until cooked through (about 15 to 20 minutes). Serve with applesauce, cooked broccoli, and a salad with oil and vinegar dressing.

Grilled Salmon Dinner

	A	B	C	D	E
Salmon steak or fillet	4 oz.	4½ oz.	5½ oz.	5½ oz.	6½ oz.
Sweet onion, large, in thick slices	1	1	1	1	1
Zucchini, 6 inches long, sliced lengthwise	1	2	2	2	2
Red bell pepper, quartered	1	1	1	1	2
Mixed salad greens	2 cups	2 cups	2 cups	2 cups	3 cups
Oil and vinegar salad dressing	1 tbsp.	1⅓ tbsp.	1½ tbsp.	1½ tbsp.	1¾ tbsp.
Peaches, fresh, or canned, drained	¾ cup	¾ cup	1 cup	1 cup	1½ cups

DIRECTIONS: Grill or broil salmon steak with garlic, salt, pepper, and lemon to taste. Slice onion, zucchini, and red pepper for outdoor grilling. Spray grill and vegetables lightly with olive oil spray to prevent sticking and grill until fork-tender and browned. Serve with salad with oil and vinegar dressing and peaches.

	MEAL PLAN PERSONAL REQUIREMENTS				
	A	B	C	D	E
Asparagus and Mushroom Omelette					
Olive oil	1 tsp.	1 tsp.	1⅓ tsp.	1⅓ tsp.	1⅓ tsp.
Mushrooms, sliced	⅔ cup	¾ cup	1 cup	1 cup	1 cup
Asparagus, sliced thin	⅔ cup	¾ cup	1 cup	1 cup	1 cup
Eggs, whole	2	2	2	2	3
Eggs, whites only	3	4	5	5	6
Parmesan cheese, grated	1½ tsp.	1½ tsp.	2 tsp.	2 tsp.	2 tsp.
Tomato, medium	1	1	1	1	1
Orange or grapefruit sections	1⅓ cups	1⅔ cups	2 cups	2 cups	2½ cups

DIRECTIONS: In a small skillet, heat olive oil and sauté mushroom pieces and asparagus. Beat eggs and cook in a nonstick pan until set. Add mushroom and asparagus mixture, fold omelette, and top with Parmesan cheese. Salt and pepper to taste. Serve with sliced tomatoes and fruit.

Family Style
Vegetable Quiche

	A	B	C	D	E
	MEAL PLAN PERSONAL REQUIREMENTS				
Quiche (recipe below)	3½ sect.	4 sect.	5 sect.	5 sect.	6 sect.
Tomato, medium	1	1	1	1	1½
Applesauce, unsweetened	⅔ cup	¾ cup	¾ cup	¾ cup	1 cup

QUICHE

1½ cup nonfat milk

2 eggs

5 egg whites

½ teaspoon salt

⅛ teaspoon pepper

1 tablespoon olive oil

½ cup chopped red onion

1 clove garlic, minced

2 cups 1-inch pieces of asparagus

½ cup chopped red or green bell pepper

1 cup ½-inch squares of extra-lean ham

3 ounces Gruyère cheese, shredded

QUICHE DIRECTIONS: Preheat oven to 325°F. In a bowl, blend nonfat milk, eggs, whites, salt, and pepper. In a skillet, heat oil and sauté onion and garlic. Add asparagus, peppers, and ham and cook until lightly browned. Transfer vegetable mixture to a nonstick 9-inch pie plate. Sprinkle with grated cheese and pour in egg mixture. Bake quiche 35 to 40 minutes or until top is golden brown. Without actually slicing, divide quiche into 12 sections to determine portions required. Then cut the appropriate serving size.

DIRECTIONS: Serve Vegetable Quiche with sliced tomatoes and applesauce.

MEAL PLAN PERSONAL REQUIREMENTS

KIDS' FAVORITE/ *Family Style*

Chicken Vegetable Soup and Salad

	A	B	C	D	E
Chicken Vegetable Soup (recipe below)	2 cups	2¼ cups	2⅔ cups	2⅔ cups	3⅓ cups
Mixed salad greens	2 cups	2½ cups	3 cups	3 cups	3 cups
Oil and vinegar salad dressing	1 tbsp.	1 tbsp.	1⅓ tbsp.	1⅓ tbsp.	1⅔ tbsp.
Black olives, large	3	4	5	5	5

CHICKEN VEGETABLE SOUP

1½ pounds chicken breast,
   cut into ¾-inch cubes

5 cups water

3 cups canned chicken broth

2 cups chopped celery

1 cup chopped onion

2 cups chopped mushroom pieces

1 cup chopped zucchini

2 ounces tomato paste

1 bay leaf

1 teaspoon salt

½ teaspoon pepper

1 clove garlic, pressed

1 cup pearl barley

CHICKEN VEGETABLE SOUP DIRECTIONS: Combine all ingredients in a Dutch oven or large pot. Bring to a boil, reduce heat, cover, and simmer for 1½ hours. Remove bay leaf before serving.

DIRECTIONS: Measure appropriate portions of Chicken Vegetable Soup using a measuring cup. Serve soup with salad, oil and vinegar dressing, and olives. If you don't like olives, double the amount of salad dressing.

	MEAL PLAN PERSONAL REQUIREMENTS				
	A	B	C	D	E

KIDS' FAVORITE/ *Family Style*

Beef Barley Soup and Salad

	A	B	C	D	E
Beef Barley Soup (recipe below)	2 cups	2¼ cups	2⅔ cups	2⅔ cups	3⅓ cups
Mixed salad greens	2 cups	2½ cups	3 cups	3 cups	3 cups
Oil and vinegar salad dressing	1 tbsp.	1 tbsp.	1⅓ tbsp.	1⅓ tbsp.	1⅔ tbsp.

BEEF BARLEY SOUP

1½ pounds boneless beef chuck

5 cups water

3 cups canned beef broth

2 cups chopped mushroom pieces

2 cups chopped celery

1 cup chopped onion

1 cup chopped zucchini

1 teaspoon salt

½ teaspoon crushed dried rosemary

½ teaspoon pepper

1 clove garlic, minced

6 ounces tomato paste

1 cup pearl barley

BEEF BARLEY SOUP DIRECTIONS: Trim meat of all visible fat and cut into ¾-inch cubes. Combine all ingredients in a Dutch oven or large pot. Bring to a full boil, reduce heat, cover, and simmer for 1½ hours.

DIRECTIONS: Measure appropriate portions of Beef Barley Soup using a measuring cup. Serve soup with salad and olive oil and vinegar dressing.

	MEAL PLAN PERSONAL REQUIREMENTS				
	A	B	C	D	E

KIDS' FAVORITE / *Family Style*

Vegetable Chili

	A	B	C	D	E
Vegetable Chili	1½ cups	1¾ cups	2 cups	2 cups	3 cups
Apple, medium	1	1	1	1	1

VEGETABLE CHILI

½ pound chicken breast, cubed

1 pound extra-lean ground beef or
   chopped sirloin

3 stalks celery, chopped

1 cup chopped red or green pepper

1 cup chopped onion

1½ cups chopped mushrooms

½ cup minced fresh parsley

1 package (1½ oz.) of chili seasoning mix

28-ounce can crushed tomatoes
   with juice

15-ounce can tomato sauce

6-ounce can tomato paste

6-ounce can water

RECIPE DIRECTIONS: Brown chicken and beef in a large Dutch oven or soup pot. Add celery, peppers, onions, mushrooms, and parsley. Cook until vegetables begin to soften. Add chili seasoning mix, tomatoes, tomato sauce, tomato paste, and water. Mix well and simmer for at least one hour. If you like your chili spicy, add ½ to 1 teaspoon crushed red pepper flakes.

DIRECTIONS: Serve chili with fresh apple slices.

	MEAL PLAN PERSONAL REQUIREMENTS				
	A	B	C	D	E
Barley Jambalaya	2½ cups	2⅔ cups	3 cups	3 cups	3⅔ cups

Family Style

Barley Jambalaya

BARLEY JAMBALAYA

2¾ tablespoons olive oil

1½ cups onion, chopped

1 cup chopped green pepper

2 cups chopped celery

2 garlic cloves, minced

14½ ounces canned diced tomatoes

4 tablespoons tomato paste

4 cups water

4 cups canned chicken broth

1 teaspoon salt

½ teaspoon dried thyme

½ teaspoon cayenne pepper

¼ teaspoon black pepper

1 bay leaf

8 drops hot pepper sauce

1 cup pearl barley

1 cup cooked ham

8 ounces cooked chicken breast,
   skin removed

12 ounces cooked shrimp, large

24 large black olives

RECIPE DIRECTIONS: Heat oil in a large soup pot. Add onion, green pepper, celery, and garlic and sauté until just beginning to brown. Add tomatoes, tomato paste, water, chicken broth, salt, thyme, cayenne pepper, black pepper, bay leaf, hot pepper sauce, and barley. Bring to a boil, then reduce heat, stir, and simmer, covered, for 1½ hours. Just prior to serving, stir in cooked ham, cooked chicken breast, shrimp, and olives. Heat through and serve.

MEAL PLAN PERSONAL REQUIREMENTS

	A	B	C	D	E
Family Style **Vegetable Lasagna**					
Vegetable Lasagna	2 slices	2¼ slices	2½ slices	2½ slices	3 slices
Apple, sliced	½ medium	¾ medium	1 medium	1 medium	1 large

VEGETABLE LASAGNA

½ large eggplant, cut into ⅛-inch-thick
    strips (for mock lasagna noodles)
1 large zucchini, cut into ⅛-inch-thick
    strips (for mock lasagna noodles)
1 tablespoon olive oil
1 cup diced onion
¼ cup diced parsley
3 cups diced mushroom stems and
    pieces, divided
1 cup diced zucchini
1 cup diced eggplant
14½ ounces canned diced tomatoes
12 ounces canned tomato paste
¼ cup water
1 teaspoon dried oregano
2 teaspoons dried basil
1½ teaspoons salt
1 cup 2% lowfat cottage cheese
15 ounces nonfat ricotta cheese
2 whole eggs
2 cups shredded part-skim
    mozzarella cheese
⅓ cup Parmesan cheese

RECIPE DIRECTIONS: Heat broiler. To make mock lasagna noodles, fill two cookie sheets with very thin lengthwise slices (approximately ⅛ inch each) of eggplant and zucchini. Place under broiler just until vegetables begin to brown, then turn and brown other side. This softens vegetables and removes some but not all of the moisture. Set aside.

Preheat oven to 375°F. Heat oil in a skillet and brown diced onion, parsley, 1 cup mushrooms, zucchini, and eggplant. Blend in tomatoes, tomato paste, water, oregano, basil, and salt to make vegetable tomato sauce. In a bowl, blend cottage cheese, ricotta cheese, and eggs. In a 10 × 13–inch baking pan, layer lasagna by placing a third of the vegetable tomato sauce, then half of the mock lasagna noodles. Top with half of the cheese mixture and 1 cup of the mushroom pieces. Sprinkle with 1 cup shredded mozzarella cheese. Add half of the remaining vegetable tomato sauce and the remaining mock lasagna noodles. Top with remaining cheese mixture, mushroom pieces, and vegetable tomato sauce. Sprinkle top with the remaining cup of mozzarella and Parmesan cheese.

DIRECTIONS: Cut lasagna into 12 even slices. Serve appropriate amount of slices for your requirements with sliced fruit.

Chapter Thirteen

FAT FLUSH DESSERTS

We believe that desserts should be part of a well-balanced diet, as long as they follow the 40-30-30 Formula. Most desserts and sweet treats are high in carbohydrates, fats, or both. But we have developed delicious desserts that contain 40 percent of calories from carbohydrates, 30 percent from protein, and 30 percent from fat.

The key to good nutrition is eating a balanced diet providing all the essential nutrients necessary to maintain the best possible state of health. Restrictive or monotonous diets deprive the dieter of the foods he or she loves, and can result in cravings and binge eating. Rather than restricting desserts, we have developed many delicious desserts to satisfy your sweet tooth. They can be used as a midafternoon snack or an after-dinner snack.

All of the dessert recipes contain 30% of calories from high quality protein sources. Each recipe has been fortified with pure whey protein powder. Pure whey protein powder is an excellent source of quality protein, has little or no taste, mixes instantly, and can be used in cooking and baking. It is derived from dairy, but is lactose free. Use a whey protein powder that is 90% pure, contains no sweeteners or flavorings, and has little or no fat or carbohydrate.

Look for a pure whey protein powder with the following nutritional profile:

PURE WHEY PROTEIN POWDER

Serving size:	1 scoop (22.2 gram size)
Calories:	80
Carbohydrate	0 grams
Protein	20 grams
Fat	0 grams

If you have trouble finding a source of pure whey protein powder, call Craig Nutraceuticals at 800-293-1683.

The following are classified as Fat Flush Formula desserts. They contain carbohydrates that are low glycemic. Rather than sugar or honey, we sweeten them with granulated fructose, a fruit sugar that is very low glycemic. Less can be used since fructose tastes sweeter than sugar. It can be purchased in health food stores in the bulk section or in bags.

THICK NEW YORK STYLE CHEESECAKE

This is the rich, New York style cheesecake you dream of.
Its delicious taste and rich texture make it a classic.

16   ounces Philadelphia Brand Fat Free Cream Cheese

16   ounces Philadelphia Light Whipped Cream Cheese

¾   cup granulated fructose

2   large eggs

1   egg white

2   teaspoons vanilla

1   cup fat free sour cream

1   tablespoon cornstarch

50   grams of pure whey protein powder

Preheat oven to 325°F. Lightly grease and flour a 9-inch springform pan.

In a large mixing bowl, beat together cream cheeses and fructose until light. Add the egg and egg white, beating thoroughly after each. Mix in the vanilla and sour cream. Add the cornstarch and whey protein powder and mix well.

Pour the mixture into the pan.

Place a pan with 1 inch of hot water in it on the bottom rack of the oven. Bake the cake at 325°F for 45 minutes on the center rack. We recommend you use a timer. Turn off the oven without opening the door and let cake cool for one hour. Let cake cool thoroughly before unmolding. It's normal for the cake to crack slightly.

To unmold, carefully run a knife between the cake and pan rim and release the sides of the springform pan. Serve plain or decorate with sliced strawberries, kiwi, or raspberries. Cake can be stored covered with plastic wrap in the refrigerator for up to 10 days, or frozen. Makes 16 servings.

Per slice: 150 calories; Grams = C-15g, P-11g, F-5g

PEANUT BUTTER CHEESECAKE

If you love peanut butter, you'll love this cheesecake.
Be sure to buy natural creamy peanut butter—the kind you have
to stir to blend the oil and peanut butter. This cake is so rich
it's guaranteed to stick to the roof of your mouth.

3	large egg whites
32	ounces Philadelphia Brand Fat Free Cream Cheese
1	cup granulated fructose
1	teaspoon vanilla
1	cup fat free sour cream
¾	cup natural full-fat creamy peanut butter
50	grams of pure whey protein powder

Preheat oven to 325°F. Lightly grease and flour a 9-inch springform pan.

In a small bowl, beat egg whites until stiff. Set aside.

In a large mixing bowl, blend the cream cheese and fructose until smooth. Add vanilla, sour cream, and peanut butter. Add whey protein powder until well blended. Gently fold the whipped egg whites into the cheese mixture until well mixed. Pour the mixture into a prepared springform pan.

Place a pan with 1 inch of hot water in it on the bottom rack of the oven. Bake the cake at 325° for 45 minutes on the center rack. Turn off the oven without opening the door, and let cake cool for 1 hour.

Cool thoroughly before unmolding.

To unmold, carefully run a knife between cake and pan rim and release the
sides of the springform pan. The cake can be stored covered with plastic wrap in the refrigerator up to 10 days, or frozen. Makes 20 servings.

Per slice: 160 calories; Grams = C-16g, P-12.5g, F-5.5g

MARBLE CHEESECAKE

This cheesecake is a showstopper and combines a striking combination of flavors with a beautiful two-color effect and a chocolate–graham cracker crust. You can swirl your own personality into every design.

2 cups 2% lowfat cottage cheese

4 ounces Philadelphia Brand ⅓ Less Fat Cream Cheese

4 ounces Philadelphia Brand Fat Free Cream Cheese

3 eggs

¾ cup granulated fructose

1 teaspoon vanilla

1½ teaspoons lemon juice

¼ teaspoon salt

40 grams of pure whey protein powder

3 tablespoons unsweetened cocoa powder

½ teaspoon instant espresso powder or instant coffee

3 tablespoons water

2 sheets chocolate graham crackers (5 × 2½ inches per sheet)

1 tablespoon butter, melted

Preheat oven to 325°F.

Spray a 9-inch round cake pan with nonstick spray and place a 9-inch parchment or waxed paper round in bottom of pan.

In a food processor, blend cottage cheese for 2 to 3 minutes until smooth.

(If using a blender, you must place the cottage cheese in a sieve or strainer and press it through to smooth the curds into a finer consistency.) Add cream cheese and blend 30 seconds. Add eggs, fructose, vanilla, lemon juice, and salt until well blended.

Add whey protein and pulse until smooth; scrape sides and blend again.

In a small bowl, mix cocoa powder, espresso powder, and water until smooth. Add 1 cup of the cheesecake batter and mix to make chocolate batter.

Pour half of the remaining cheesecake batter into the prepared pan. Slowly pour the chocolate batter into center of the pan, then add the remaining plain batter in center of the chocolate. This should have formed a chocolate ring. Using a knife, make circular strokes to marbleize the batter.

Place a pan with 1 inch of hot water on the bottom rack of the oven. Bake cake at 325°F for 40 to 50 minutes on the center rack until the center of the cake barely jiggles when cake is shaken.

While the cake is still hot, carefully run a knife between the cake and pan rim, then refrigerate uncovered until cool, about two hours. Unmold the cake and remove the parchment paper from bottom. Return to a serving platter.

Combine graham cracker crumbs and melted butter. Using a knife, press the crumbs around the sides of the cake. Cover and refrigerate for at least 6 to 12 hours before serving. Cake can be stored covered with plastic wrap for up to 10 days, or frozen. Makes 12 servings.

Per slice: 160 calories; Grams = C-17g, P-12g, F-5g

CHOCOLATE CHEESECAKE

This cheesecake combines an elegant visual appeal
with a distinctive, delicious, full chocolate taste.
Now chocolate lovers can indulge without the bulge.

- 2 cups 2% lowfat cottage cheese
- 4 ounces Philadelphia Brand ⅓ Less Cream Cheese
- 4 ounces Philadelphia Brand Fat Free Cream Cheese
- 2 eggs
- 2 egg whites
- ½ cup granulated fructose
- 40 grams of pure whey protein powder
- ¾ cup cocoa powder
- ¼ cup nonfat milk
- 1 teaspoon vanilla
- 1½ ounces semisweet chocolate
- 1½ sheets of chocolate graham crackers (5 × 2½ inches per sheet)
- ½ tablespoon butter, melted

Preheat oven to 325°F.

Spray an 8-inch cake pan with nonstick spray and place an 8-inch parchment round or waxed paper in the bottom of pan.

In a food processor, blend the cottage cheese for 2 to 3 minutes until smooth. (If using a blender, you must place the cottage cheese in a sieve or strainer and press it through to smooth the curds into a finer consistency.) Add cream cheese and blend 30 seconds. Add eggs, egg whites, and fructose and mix until well blended.

In a small bowl, combine whey protein powder with cocoa powder. Add to cheese mixture with nonfat milk and vanilla and blend well.

Microwave the semisweet chocolate in a glass cup until melted, then scrape it into the cheese mixture and blend. Pour the mixture into a prepared pan.

Place a pan with 1 inch of hot water in it on the bottom rack of the oven. Bake the cake on the center rack for 40 to 45 minutes at 325°F. The center should barely jiggle when cake is shaken.

While still hot, carefully run a knife between cake and pan rim, then refrigerate uncovered until cool, about 2 hours. Unmold cake and remove parchment paper from bottom. Return to a serving platter.

Combine graham cracker crumbs and melted butter. Using a knife, press crumbs around the side of the cake. Cover and refrigerate for at least 6 to 12 hours before serving. Serve plain or decorate with fresh raspberries or dust with cocoa powder for an elegant touch. Makes 12 slices.

Per slice: 160 calories; Grams = C-17g, P-12g, F-5g

KIDS' FAVORITE
RICH CHOCOLATE PUDDING

Everyone from kids to seniors will love this rich and creamy chocolate pudding. They won't believe something that tastes this great is made from tofu.

10½	ounces lowfat silken tofu
½	teaspoon vanilla
1½	tablespoons natural creamy peanut butter
2	tablespoons cocoa powder
2½	tablespoons granulated fructose
10	grams of pure whey protein powder

In a small food processor, blend tofu on high until creamy. Add vanilla and peanut butter and blend for 30 seconds.

Add cocoa powder and fructose; mix gently with a spatula, then blend for 1 more minute, opening processor to scrape the sides.

Mix in the protein powder and blend for 1 more minute, scraping sides if needed.

Measure equal portions into 4 small cup servings and cover with plastic wrap before refrigerating. Makes 4 servings. This recipe can be doubled if using a full-size food processor.

Per serving: 130 calories; Grams = C-12.5g, P-9.75g, F-4.5g

KIDS' FAVORITE
VANILLA CUSTARD

This recipe makes 6 little cups of velvety
smooth vanilla custard. They are an
elegant little ending to any dinner party.

2 cups 2% lowfat milk

3 whole eggs

2 egg whites

⅛ teaspoon salt

¼ cup granulated fructose

1½ teaspoon vanilla

15 grams of pure whey protein powder

Preheat oven to 325°F.

In a medium saucepan, heat milk until just steaming.

In a mixing bowl with a pour spout, whisk eggs and whites, salt, fructose, and vanilla. Slowly add steaming milk, whisking continuously. Add whey protein powder and blend well.

Bake in a water bath: Line the bottom of a glass or metal cake or roasting pan with several sheets of paper towels. Place 6 ramekin custard cups (6 ounces each) in the pan and fill them with vanilla custard mixture. Carefully pour hot water into the pan to reach half to two-thirds of the way up the sides of the custard dishes. Very carefully, place the pan in the center of the oven. Bake at 325°F for 35 minutes. Carefully remove custards from oven and let sit for 10 minutes to cool slightly before removing custard cups from water bath. Chill in refrigerator for two hours, and serve cold. Makes 6 servings.

Per serving: 125 calories; Grams = C-12.5g, P-9.5g, F-4g

Part Three

THE FORMULA
FOR LIFE

Chapter Fourteen

YOUR MAINTENANCE PLAN

You have completed the 21-Day Fat Flush Formula—now what? You have a few options. You can continue to follow the Fat Flush Formula Meals exclusively until you lose all of the weight you want and have reached your goal weight. Many of our clients have lost more than 100 pounds in a year on the Fat Flush Formula. You can also choose to use Regular Formula Meals or combine the two plans. Regular Formula Meals contain the 40-30-30 ratio, but the carbohydrates they contain are a combination of low, medium, and high glycemic carbohydrates, and offer a wider variety of foods. Use Regular Formula Meals to continue weight loss and for the Formula for Life maintenance plan.

If you experience a "plateau," always return to the Fat Flush Formula meals for a few days or a week. The Fat Flush Formula meals accelerate fat loss with tighter controls on blood sugar levels. Once you reach your ideal weight, your body generally finds its set point and will maintain that weight. If weight loss continues, you may find it necessary to use only

Regular Formula Meals or move to the next larger meal plan. The additional calories will stop any unwanted weight loss.

By no means should you feel that you must prepare every one of the Regular Formula Meals. Use the meals you like and you will see the best results. It doesn't matter if you find a few favorites and eat those same few meals over and over. One of our clients who used to be overweight ate a bowl of cereal for breakfast and a burger and fries for lunch every day. After following the Formula and reaching his ideal weight, he now eats a 40-30-30 smoothie or an egg burrito for breakfast, a turkey sandwich or Wendy's chili for lunch, and a 40-30-30 Nutrition Bar as a 4:00 P.M. snack. His dinners vary, but it's easier for him to eat from a limited selection of foods that he knows are balanced and make him feel good. His goal was to change the meals he ate that made him fat and eat meals to keep him fit. He was surprised to discover that by eating meals that stabilize blood sugar levels, he not only lost excess body fat—his energy levels improved along with focus and concentration.

Once you understand how a balanced diet can help you control the hormones that burn fat and improve health, energy, and concentration, you will have discovered the simple but powerful Formula for Life.

WHAT MEAL PLAN IS RIGHT FOR YOU?

The Formula personalized meal plans have been designed for your individual 40-30-30 requirements. Your gender, body weight, and activity level determine the overall amount of food and calories you need daily to maximize the burning of stored fat for energy. There are five different-size personalized plans for you to choose from.

When choosing the plan, use your current actual weight, not your goal weight. For example, if you are a woman weighing 195 pounds and moderately active, choose the C plan. When your weight drops to 180 pounds, switch to the B plan.

Review the Formula Meal Plan Selection Chart on the next page to choose the correct size plan for your requirements.

If you are an elite athlete, training more than 10 hours per week and competitive in your sport, you will certainly require more calories than a noncompetitive person the same size. Highly trained muscles have greater energy requirements. Review the Formula Meal Plan Selection Chart for Elite Athletes (page 137) to choose the correct size plan for your needs.

THE FORMULA
MEAL PLAN SELECTION CHART

WOMEN

Activity Level	Low–Moderate	Medium–High
Hours of Exercise per Week	Exercise 0–4 hours per week	Exercise 5–10 hours per week
Current Body Weight	*Use Meal Planner*	*Use Meal Planner*
Under 140	A	B
141–180	B	C
181–200+	C	D

MEN

Activity Level	Low–Moderate	Medium–High
Hours of Exercise per Week	Exercise 0–4 hours per week	Exercise 5–10 hours per week
Current Body Weight	*Use Meal Planner*	*Use Meal Planner*
Under 140	B	C
141–180	C	D
181–250+	C	D

Your Personalized Meal Plan is _____

THE FORMULA
MEAL PLAN SELECTION CHART FOR ELITE ATHLETES

FEMALE ELITE ATHLETES

Current Body Weight	Train 10 or more hours per week
Under 140	C
141–180	D
180 and over	E

MALE ELITE ATHLETES

Current Body Weight	Train 10 or more hours per week
Under 140	C
141–180	D
180 and over	E

MACRONUTRIENT CHART

Listed below you will find the total grams of carbohydrate, protein, fat, and calories listed for each meal plan. The meal planners have been tailored for individual requirements based on gender, weight, and activity levels. To determine which meal planner is right for you, refer to the Meal Plan Selection Chart. Each meal and snack contains the 40-30-30 ratio, which provides 40 percent of its *total calories* from carbohydrates, 30 percent from protein, and 30 percent from fat.

Personal Meal Plan	A	B	C	D	E
BREAKFAST					
Carbohydrate grams	20	20	33	47	53
Protein grams	15	15	25	35	40
Fat grams	6	6	11	13	18
Calories	194	194	331	445	534
LUNCH					
Carbohydrate grams	27	40	40	53	66
Protein grams	20	30	30	40	50
Fat grams	9	14	14	18	22
Calories	269	406	406	534	662
SNACKS					
Carbohydrate grams	20	20	20	20	40
Protein grams	15	15	15	15	30
Fat grams	6	6	6	6	12
Calories	194	194	194	194	388
DINNER					
Carbohydrate grams	40	47	53	53	66
Protein grams	30	35	40	40	50
Fat grams	14	15	18	18	22
Calories	406	463	534	534	662

Personal Meal Plan	A	B	C	D	E
DAILY TOTALS					
Carbohydrate grams	106	126	146	173	226
Protein grams	80	95	110	130	170
Fat grams	35	42	48	57	75
Calories	1,063	1,257	1,465	1,707	2,246

WHAT SHOULD YOU DRINK?

Because water is so vital to good health and helps to maximize the fat burning process, it is always your best choice when following the Formula. Refer to chapter one to determine your approximate water requirements.

Listed below are several examples of what to drink when following the Formula:

- Try to drink eight to twelve ounces of water at the start and end of each day.
- Drink six additional eight- to twelve-ounce glasses of water throughout the day, for a total of eight glasses of water or other appropriate beverages per day.
- Avoid or limit sugar and caffeinated beverages (especially beverages that contain sugar). Appropriate sugar-free and decaffeinated beverages include: water, mineral water, herbal teas, green tea, caffeine-free diet soft drinks, and decaffeinated coffee, tea, or hot water with lemon.

- If drinking fruit juice, consume only small amounts and dilute the juice with extra water.

- If you drink vegetable juice or if you use a juicer, use primarily lower glycemic vegetables such as parsley, peppers, spinach, broccoli, cabbage, and celery and reduce your consumption of high glycemic vegetables such as carrots, beets, and apples.

- A popular 40-30-30 beverage is a lowfat, decaffeinated latte, hot or iced. A latte is a coffee drink that contains steamed milk and a shot of espresso. Lowfat milk is close to the 40-30-30 ratio naturally, and with a shot of decaffeinated espresso is a delicious occasional treat for coffee lovers. You can make a mocha latte by adding unsweetened cocoa powder and a little artificial sweetener. Note: Use artificial sweeteners in moderation.

- 1% lowfat milk meets the 40-30-30 criteria naturally and can be used as part of your meal or as a snack.

- Because alcohol converts into sugar, always include a little lowfat protein with an alcoholic beverage.

Chapter Fifteen

REGULAR BREAKFASTS

The next few chapters will provide you with recipes for delicious meals that follow the Regular Formula. Before you dive right in, please read the following information about one of the ingredients called for in some of the recipes.

PURE WHEY PROTEIN POWDER

Whey protein is the newest generation of protein powder and contains an impressive amino acid profile. It is easy to digest, mixes instantly, and has no chalky aftertaste. It is basically tasteless and works extremely well when used in certain recipes.

Although there are a lot of different types of protein powders out there (made from soy, casein, or egg proteins, to name a few), we feel that whey protein is the best type to use.

When shopping for a whey protein powder, look for one that contains pure protein and nothing else. Many protein powders contain carbohydrates, fat, and artificial sweeteners and flavors.

The very best whey protein powders are 90% pure protein. To determine the percentage of purity of a protein powder, take the total serving size (in grams) and multiply by .90. The number you get should be the same as the total grams of protein listed in the nutritional information on the label. There should be one gram or less per serving of carbohydrates and fat.

The whey protein powder we use in our recipes has (per 22.2-gram scoop) 80 calories, zero grams of carbohydrates, zero grams of fat, and 20 grams of protein.

When we call for pure whey protein powder in our recipes, the measurement we use is grams. Each container of powder comes with a scoop, which equals about 20 grams of protein. Please use the following chart to aid you in measuring the grams of whey protein powder for each recipe. (For example, a quarter-scoop of powder contains 5 grams of protein.)

Pure whey protein powder can usually be found in health food stores. If you have trouble finding it, call Craig Nutraceuticals, Inc., at 800-293-1683.

Ask for Pure WPI by Bioplex Nutrition.

Scoop	Grams
1/4	5
1/3	7
1/2	10
2/3	13
3/4	15
1	20

MEAL PLAN PERSONAL REQUIREMENTS

KIDS' FAVORITE
Banana Walnut Smoothie

	A	B	C	D	E
Banana, medium	⅓	⅓	⅔	1	1
Milk, 1% lowfat	½ cup	½ cup	⅔ cup	1 cup	1⅓ cups
Granulated fructose	1 tsp.	1 tsp.	1 tsp.	1 tsp.	2 tsp.
Pure whey protein powder	10 grams	10 grams	15 grams	20 grams	25 grams
Walnuts, chopped	1 tbsp.	1 tbsp.	2 tbsp.	2¾ tbsp.	3⅓ tbsp.

DIRECTIONS: Combine all ingredients in a blender and process until smooth. Use frozen peeled bananas for a thicker smoothie.

KIDS' FAVORITE
Cocoa Banana Smoothie

	A	B	C	D	E
Banana, medium	⅓	⅓	½	⅔	1
Milk, 1% lowfat	½ cup	½ cup	⅔ cup	1 cup	1 cup
Cocoa powder, unsweetened	2 tsp.	2 tsp.	2 tsp.	2 tsp.	2 tsp.
Pure whey protein powder	10 grams	10 grams	15 grams	20 grams	25 grams
Granulated fructose	1 tsp.	1 tsp.	1½ tsp.	2½ tsp.	2 tsp.
Peanut butter, natural	2 tsp.	2 tsp.	1 tbsp.	1½ tbsp.	1¾ tbsp.

DIRECTIONS: Blend all ingredients in a blender until smooth. Use frozen peeled bananas for a thicker smoothie.

KIDS' FAVORITE
Strawberry-Banana Smoothie

	A	B	C	D	E
Strawberries	½ cup	½ cup	¾ cup	1 cup	1 cup
Banana, medium	¼	¼	½	¾	1
Water	½ cup	½ cup	¾ cup	1 cup	1 cup
Granulated fructose	2 tsp.	2 tsp.	2 tsp.	1 tbsp.	1 tbsp.
Pure whey protein powder	13 grams	13 grams	20 grams	30 grams	33 grams
Almonds, sliced	1⅔ tbsp.	1⅔ tbsp.	2⅔ tbsp.	3¾ tbsp.	¼ cup+2 tsp.

DIRECTIONS: Blend all ingredients in a blender until smooth. Use frozen strawberries and bananas for a thicker smoothie.

	MEAL PLAN PERSONAL REQUIREMENTS				
	A	B	C	D	E

KIDS' FAVORITE

Breakfast Pizza

	A	B	C	D	E
English muffin	½	½	¾	1	1½
Canadian bacon	1½ oz.	1½ oz.	2 oz.	3 oz.	4 oz.
Pineapple rings, canned, drained	1 ring	1 ring	1½ rings	2 rings	2 rings
Mozzarella cheese, part skim milk, grated	½ oz.	½ oz.	1 oz.	1 oz.	1½ oz.

DIRECTIONS: Lightly toast English muffin halves. Top with Canadian bacon, pineapple, and cheese. Place under the broiler until cheese melts and begins to brown.

Bagel Sandwich

	A	B	C	D	E
Bagel, plain, wheat, or oat bran, 3½-inch diameter	½	½	¾	1	1¼
Cream cheese, Philadelphia Brand lowfat	2½ tbsp.	2½ tbsp.	3½ tbsp.	5 tbsp.	6 tbsp.
or					
Cream cheese, full fat	1¼ tbsp.	1¼ tbsp.	1¾ tbsp.	2½ tbsp.	3 tbsp.
Lean deli meat (turkey, chicken, or roast beef)	2 oz.	2 oz.	3 oz.	4½ oz.	5 oz.

DIRECTIONS: Spread plain or toasted bagel halves with cream cheese and top with sliced deli meat. Note: Choose amount from either lowfat or full fat cream cheese.

	MEAL PLAN PERSONAL REQUIREMENTS				
	A	B	C	D	E
Bagel, Lox, and Cream Cheese					
Bagel, plain, wheat, or oat bran, 3½-inch diameter	½	½	¾	1	1¼
Cream cheese, Philadelphia Brand lowfat	1½ tbsp.	1½ tbsp.	2⅔ tbsp.	3¾ tbsp.	4½ tbsp.
or					
Cream cheese, full fat	¾ tbsp.	¾ tbsp.	1⅓ tbsp.	2 tbsp.	2¼ tbsp.
Lox	2 oz.	2 oz.	3 oz.	4 oz.	5 oz.
Onion slices	1	1	1½	2	2
Fresh dill (optional)	⅛ tsp.	⅛ tsp.	¼ tsp.	¼ tsp.	½ tsp.

DIRECTIONS: Spread bagel halves with cream cheese. Top with lox, onion slices, and fresh dill. Note: Choose amount from either lowfat or full fat cream cheese.

KIDS' FAVORITE

One-Eyed Sandwich					
Bread, whole grain	1 slice	1 slice	2 slices	3 slices	4 slices
Whipped butter	½ tsp.	½ tsp.	½ tsp.	1 tsp.	1 tsp.
Eggs, whole	1	1	2	2	3
Eggs, whites only	2	2	2	4	4
Orange, medium size, quartered	½	½	¾	1	1

DIRECTIONS: Remove and discard a 3-inch-diameter circle from the center of bread slices. Lightly butter the remaining edges and place in a hot nonstick pan. Break eggs and whites in center and cook until set. Turn to brown both sides. Salt and pepper to taste. Serve with quartered orange slices.

	MEAL PLAN PERSONAL REQUIREMENTS				
	A	B	C	D	E

KIDS' FAVORITE
Egg and Cheese Burrito

	A	B	C	D	E
Eggs, whole	1	1	1	2	2
Eggs, whites only	2	2	3	3	4
Tortilla, flour, 7- to 8-inch diameter	1	1	2	2	2½
Cheddar cheese, lowfat, shredded	2 tsp.	2 tsp.	3 tbsp.	2 tbsp.	2½ tbsp.
Sour cream, lowfat	2 tsp.	2 tsp.	2 tbsp.	2 tbsp.	2½ tbsp.
Salsa	1 tbsp.	1 tbsp.	2 tbsp.	3 tbsp.	3 tbsp.

DIRECTIONS: Scramble eggs and whites in a nonstick pan. Place cooked eggs, shredded cheese, sour cream, and salsa in warmed tortilla. Roll and eat.

KIDS' FAVORITE
Breakfast Burrito with Chicken

	A	B	C	D	E
Corn tortilla, 5-inch diameter	1	1	2	2	3
Cooked chicken breast, sliced	2 oz.	2 oz.	3 oz.	4 oz.	5 oz.
Sour cream, lowfat	1 tbsp.	1 tbsp.	2 tbsp.	2 tbsp.	2 tbsp.
Salsa	1 tbsp.	1 tbsp.	2 tbsp.	2 tbsp.	2 tbsp.
Avocado, medium, slices	⅛ slice	⅛ slice	¼ slice	¼ slice	⅓ slice
Black olives, large, sliced	2	2	2	6	6
Orange, medium size	⅓	⅓	⅓	¾	¾

DIRECTIONS: Warm tortilla and chicken. Place chicken slices on tortilla with sour cream, salsa, avocado, and black olives. Roll and eat with fresh orange sections.

MEAL PLAN PERSONAL REQUIREMENTS

Scrambled Eggs and Toast

	A	B	C	D	E
Eggs, whole	1	1	1	2	2
Eggs, whites only	2	2	4	5	6
Bread, reduced calorie whole wheat, toasted	1 slice	1 slice	2 slices	2 slices	2 slices
Whipped butter	1 tsp.	1 tsp.	2 tsp.	2 tsp.	1 tbsp.
Preserves, any flavor	1 tsp.	1 tsp.	1 tsp.	2 tsp.	2 tsp.
Orange, medium size	½	½	½	1	1½

DIRECTIONS: Scramble eggs and whites in a nonstick pan. Spread toast with whipped butter and preserves. Serve eggs and toast with fresh orange sections.

Vegetable Omelette

	A	B	C	D	E
Eggs, whole	1	1	2	2	3
Eggs, whites only	2	2	3	5	5
Olive oil spray	spray	spray	spray	spray	spray
Red potatoes, cooked	⅓ cup	⅓ cup	½ cup	⅔ cup	¾ cup
Onion, diced	1 tbsp.	1 tbsp.	2 tbsp.	2 tbsp.	2 tbsp.
Green bell pepper, diced	1 tbsp.	1 tbsp.	2 tbsp.	2 tbsp.	2 tbsp.
Sour cream, lowfat	1 tbsp.	1 tbsp.	1 tbsp.	2 tbsp.	2 tbsp.
Strawberries, fresh sliced	⅓ cup	⅓ cup	⅔ cup	1⅓ cups	1⅓ cups

DIRECTIONS: Beat eggs and whites. Heat a pan sprayed with olive oil and sauté cooked potatoes, onion, and green pepper until just beginning to brown. Heat a nonstick omelette pan lightly sprayed with olive oil and cook egg mixture until almost set. Add vegetables and sour cream and fold omelette. Serve with fresh strawberries.

| | MEAL PLAN PERSONAL REQUIREMENTS | | | | |
	A	B	C	D	E

French Toast and Canadian Bacon

	A	B	C	D	E
Eggs, whole	1	1	1	1	2
Eggs, whites only	1	1	1	1	1
Milk, 1% lowfat	1 tbsp.	1 tbsp.	2 tbsp.	3 tbsp.	3 tbsp.
Vanilla	¼ tsp.	¼ tsp.	½ tsp.	½ tsp.	½ tsp.
Salt	dash	dash	dash	dash	dash
Bread, reduced calorie whole wheat	1½ slices	1½ slices	2 slices	3 slices	4 slices
Powdered sugar	½ tsp.	½ tsp.	½ tsp.	½ tsp.	1 tsp.
Maple syrup	1 tsp.	1 tsp.	2 tsp.	2½ tsp.	2½ tsp.
Canadian bacon	¾ oz.	¾ oz.	1½ oz.	2¾ oz.	2¾ oz.

DIRECTIONS: In a medium bowl, blend eggs and whites, milk, vanilla, and salt. Place bread slices in the egg mixture, allowing them to absorb it all, and cook on both sides in a nonstick pan until brown. Top with powdered sugar and syrup and serve with heated Canadian bacon slices.

Yogurt Plus

	A	B	C	D	E
Yogurt, nonfat with fruit, any flavor	⅓ cup	⅓ cup	½ cup	¾ cup	1 cup
Cottage cheese, 2% lowfat	⅓ cup	⅓ cup	½ cup	¾ cup	1 cup
Granola	1 tbsp.	1 tbsp.	1½ tbsp.	1 tbsp.	1½ tbsp.
Almonds, sliced	1 tbsp.	1 tbsp.	1½ tbsp.	1½ tbsp.	2½ tbsp.

DIRECTIONS: Combine nonfat fruit yogurt with cottage cheese. Top with granola and almonds.

MEAL PLAN PERSONAL REQUIREMENTS

	A	B	C	D	E

KIDS' FAVORITE
Banana Split Deluxe

	A	B	C	D	E
Banana, large	⅓	⅓	½	¾	1
Cottage cheese, 2% lowfat	½ cup	½ cup	¾ cup	1 cup	1⅓ cups
Pineapple chunks, drained	¼ cup	¼ cup	⅓ cup	½ cup	⅔ cup
Strawberries, fresh	¼ cup	¼ cup	⅓ cup	½ cup	⅔ cup
Almonds, sliced	1⅓ tbsp.	1⅓ tbsp.	2 tbsp.	3 tbsp.	3⅓ tbsp.
Cinnamon	dash	dash	dash	dash	dash

DIRECTIONS: Place horizontally sliced banana in a bowl. Top with cottage cheese, pineapple, and strawberries. Sprinkle with almonds and cinnamon.

KIDS' FAVORITE
Cold Cheese and Fruit Pizza

	A	B	C	D	E
English muffin	½	½	¾	1	1½
Cottage cheese, 2% lowfat	⅓ cup	⅓ cup	⅔ cup	¾ cup	1 cup
Strawberries, fresh, large	1 whole	1 whole	2 whole	2 whole	2 whole
Almonds, sliced	1⅓ tbsp.	1⅓ tbsp.	2 tbsp.	2¾ tbsp.	3½ tbsp.
Honey	¼ tsp.	¼ tsp.	½ tsp.	1 tsp.	1 tsp.

DIRECTIONS: Toast English muffin halves. Top with cottage cheese, sliced strawberries, and sliced almonds, and drizzle with honey.

Cereal with Protein Powder

	A	B	C	D	E
Milk, 1% lowfat	⅓ cup	⅓ cup	½ cup	½ cup	¾ cup
Pure whey protein powder	10 grams	10 grams	15 grams	20 grams	25 grams
Cereal (Kellogg's Shredded Wheat)	½ cup	½ cup	⅔ cup	1 cup	1¼ cups
Nuts, chopped (almonds, pecans, or walnuts)	1⅔ tbsp.	1⅔ tbsp.	2½ tbsp.	3½ tbsp.	¼ cup

DIRECTIONS: In a bowl, blend milk with whey protein powder. Add cereal and nuts.

MEAL PLAN PERSONAL REQUIREMENTS

Cereal with Eggs

	A	B	C	D	E
Cereal (Kellogg's Shredded Wheat)	½ cup	½ cup	⅔ cup	1 cup	1 cup
Milk, 1% lowfat	½ cup	½ cup	½ cup	¾ cup	¾ cup
Strawberries, fresh, sliced	¼ cup	¼ cup	¼ cup	¼ cup	½ cup
Almonds, sliced	1 tsp.	1 tsp.	1 tbsp.	2 tbsp.	1½ tbsp.
Eggs, whole	1	1	1	1	2
Eggs, whites only	2	2	3	4	4

DIRECTIONS: In a bowl, combine cereal and milk and add sliced strawberries and almonds. Serve with cooked eggs and whites, scrambled, poached, or hard-boiled.

Cereal and Canadian Bacon

	A	B	C	D	E
Cereal (Kellogg's All-Bran)	⅓ cup	⅓ cup	⅔ cup	¾ cup	1 cup
Milk, 1% lowfat	½ cup	½ cup	½ cup	¾ cup	¾ cup
Almonds, sliced	1 tsp.	1 tsp.	2 tsp.	1 tbsp.	1 tbsp.
Canadian bacon, sliced	1½ oz.	1½ oz.	2½ oz.	3 oz.	4 oz.

DIRECTIONS: Combine cereal, milk, and almonds in a bowl. Serve with heated Canadian bacon.

Cereal with Soy Milk

	A	B	C	D	E
Soy milk, plain	⅓ cup	⅓ cup	½ cup	½ cup	½ cup
Pure whey protein powder	10 grams	10 grams	13 grams	20 grams	25 grams
Cereal (Kellogg's All-Bran)	⅓ cup	⅓ cup	½ cup	⅔ cup	¾ cup
Almonds, sliced	1½ tbsp.	1½ tbsp.	2½ tbsp.	3½ tbsp.	¼ cup
Strawberries, fresh, large	2	2	2	2	2

DIRECTIONS: Blend soy milk with pure whey protein powder in a bowl. Add cereal and top with almonds and sliced strawberries.

MEAL PLAN PERSONAL REQUIREMENTS

Hot Cereal and Cream

	A	B	C	D	E
Oatmeal, cooked	½ cup	½ cup	¾ cup	1 cup	1⅓ cups
Cottage cheese, 2% lowfat	⅓ cup	⅓ cup	⅔ cup	¾ cup	1 cup
Brown sugar	1 tsp.	1 tsp.	1½ tsp.	2 tsp.	2 tsp.
Whipped butter	½ tsp.	½ tsp.	1 tsp.	1½ tsp.	1½ tsp.
Milk, 1% lowfat	3 tbsp.	3 tbsp.	3 tbsp.	¼ cup	¼ cup
Almonds, sliced	2 tsp.	2 tsp.	1 tbsp.	1⅓ tbsp.	1¾ tbsp.

DIRECTIONS: Blend cottage cheese into hot oatmeal and top with brown sugar, butter, milk, and almonds. Cottage cheese melts and becomes very creamy. It can also be served on the side.

KIDS' FAVORITE

40-30-30 Nutrition Bar

	A	B	C	D	E
40-30-30 Nutrition Bar, any flavor	1	1	1	2	2
Milk, 1% lowfat	0	0	8 oz.	8 oz.	12 oz.

DIRECTIONS: When using a 40-30-30 Nutrition Bar as a breakfast meal replacement, 1 bar with water, coffee, or tea is appropriate for the A or B plan. If you are following the C, D, or E plan, one bar is not enough. Have 1 to 2 bars with lowfat milk and add water, coffee, or tea.

KIDS' FAVORITE

40-30-30 Shake Mix

	A	B	C	D	E
40-30-30 Shake Mix, any flavor	1 packet	1 packet	1 packet	2 packets	2 packets
Water	8 oz.	8 oz.	4 oz.	8 oz.	8 oz.
Milk, 1% lowfat	0	0	4 oz.	8 oz.	12 oz.

DIRECTIONS: When using a 40-30-30 Shake Mix as a breakfast meal replacement, 1 packet with water is appropriate for the A or B plan. If you are following the C, D, or E plan, one packet is not enough. Have 1 to 2 packets with water and lowfat milk. For a thicker shake, use a blender and add ice cubes for part of the water.

Chapter Sixteen

REGULAR LUNCHES

	MEAL PLAN PERSONAL REQUIREMENTS				
	A	B	C	D	E

KIDS' FAVORITE
Banana Peanut Butter Smoothie

	A	B	C	D	E
Banana, medium	⅔	1	1	1⅓	1¾
Milk, 1% lowfat	⅔ cup	¾ cup	¾ cup	1 cup	1 cup
Peanut butter, natural	2½ tsp.	1⅓ tbsp.	1⅓ tbsp.	1¾ tbsp.	2⅓ tbsp.
Pure whey protein powder	10 grams	20 grams	20 grams	25 grams	33 grams

DIRECTIONS: Combine all ingredients in a blender and process until smooth. Use frozen bananas for a thicker smoothie.

KIDS' FAVORITE
Fruit Smoothie

	A	B	C	D	E
Banana, medium	⅓ cup	½ cup	½ cup	⅔ cup	¾ cup
Peaches, frozen	½ cup	¾ cup	¾ cup	1 cup	1½ cups
Water	½ cup	¾ cup	¾ cup	1 cup	1⅓ cups
Pure whey protein powder	15 grams	25 grams	25 grams	30 grams	40 grams
Almonds, sliced	2⅓ tbsp.	3½ tbsp.	3½ tbsp.	¼ cup+2 tsp.	⅓ cup

DIRECTIONS: Blend all ingredients in a blender until smooth. Use frozen bananas for a thicker smoothie.

MEAL PLAN PERSONAL REQUIREMENTS

	A	B	C	D	E

Tropical Breeze Smoothie

	A	B	C	D	E
Pineapple, fresh or canned in natural juices	1⅓ cups	2 cups	2 cups	2⅔ cups	3⅓ cups
Water with ice cubes	½ cup	½ cup	½ cup	⅔ cup	¾ cup
Pure whey protein powder	20 grams	30 grams	30 grams	40 grams	50 grams
Macadamia nuts, chopped	1⅓ tbsp.	2 tbsp.	2 tbsp.	2⅔ tbsp.	3⅓ tbsp.

DIRECTIONS: Blend all ingredients in a blender until smooth.

Gene's Power Pack

	A	B	C	D	E
Banana, medium	⅓ cup	½ cup	½ cup	¾ cup	1 cup
Strawberries, frozen	1 cup	1 cup	1 cup	1½ cups	1⅔ cups
Milk, 1% lowfat	½ cup	1 cup	1 cup	1 cup	1½ cups
Pure whey protein powder	15 grams	20 grams	20 grams	30 grams	35 grams
Bee pollen	1 tsp.	1 tsp.	1 tsp.	1½ tsp.	1½ tsp.
Emer'gen-C™ packet	1 packet	1 packet	1 packet	1 packet	1 packet
Flax oil	½ tbsp.	¾ tbsp.	¾ tbsp.	1¼ tbsp.	1⅓ tbsp.

DIRECTIONS: Combine all ingredients in a blender and process until smooth. Use frozen bananas for a thicker smoothie. Bee pollen, Emer'gen-C™, and flax oil can be found in health food stores.

Deli-Salad Pita Pocket

	A	B	C	D	E
Deli-style tuna or chicken salad with full-fat mayonnaise	4 oz.	5 oz.	5 oz.	7 oz.	9 oz.
Pita bread, wheat or white	½	¾	¾	1	1
Apple	½ medium	½ medium	½ medium	1 medium	1 large

DIRECTIONS: Purchase tuna or chicken salad made with full-fat mayonnaise from a deli. Place in pita pocket and serve with fruit.

MEAL PLAN PERSONAL REQUIREMENTS

Egg Salad in Pita Pocket

	A	B	C	D	E
Eggs, whole	1	2	2	2	3
Eggs, whites only	2	4	4	6	7
Pickle relish, sweet or dill	1 tbsp.	1⅓ tbsp.	1⅓ tbsp.	1½ tbsp.	3 tbsp.
Celery, diced	1 tbsp.	2 tbsp.	2 tbsp.	2 tbsp.	3 tbsp.
Mayonnaise, reduced-fat	1¾ tbsp.	1¾ tbsp.	1¾ tbsp.	2¾ tbsp.	3 tbsp.
Mustard, prepared	1 tsp.	2 tsp.	2 tsp.	2 tsp.	1 tbsp.
Pita bread, wheat or white	½	¾	¾	1	1½
Grapes	⅓ cup	½ cup	½ cup	½ cup	½ cup

DIRECTIONS: Hard-boil eggs, cool, peel, and discard some of the yolks. Dice eggs and mix with pickle relish, celery, mayonnaise, and mustard. Season with salt and pepper to taste. Place egg salad in pita pocket and serve with grapes.

Soft Chicken Tacos

	A	B	C	D	E
Corn tortilla, 5- to 6-inch diameter	2	3	3	4	5
Sour cream, lowfat	2 tbsp.	3 tbsp.	3 tbsp.	4 tbsp.	4 tbsp.
Cooked chicken breast, shredded	2 oz.	3 oz.	3 oz.	4 oz.	5 oz.
Salsa	2 tbsp.	3 tbsp.	3 tbsp.	3 tbsp.	4 tbsp.
Cabbage, shredded	½ cup	⅔ cup	⅔ cup	¾ cup	1 cup
Cheddar cheese, shredded, full-fat	2½ tbsp.	¼ cup	¼ cup	⅓ cup	⅓ cup+1 tbsp.

DIRECTIONS: Place sour cream, chicken, salsa, shredded cabbage, and cheddar cheese on a warmed soft corn tortilla. Fold and eat.

MEAL PLAN PERSONAL REQUIREMENTS

Bagel Sandwich

	A	B	C	D	E
Bagel, plain, wheat, or oat bran, 3½-inch diameter	½	½	½	1	1½
Avocado, medium, mashed	¼ slice	⅓ slice	⅓ slice	⅓ slice	½ slice
Lean deli meat (turkey, chicken, or roast beef)	2 oz.	3½ oz.	3½ oz.	4 oz.	4 oz.
Swiss cheese, lowfat	1 oz.	1 oz.	1 oz.	1½ oz.	2 oz.
Strawberries, sliced	½ cup	1½ cups	1½ cups	1 cup	1 cup

DIRECTIONS: Spread bagel halves with avocado and top with deli meat and cheese. Serve with sliced strawberries.

KIDS' FAVORITE

Grilled Ham and Cheese

	A	B	C	D	E
Bread, reduced-calorie wheat or white	2	3	3	4	5
Whipped butter	2 tsp.	1 tbsp.	1 tbsp.	1⅓ tbsp.	1½ tbsp.
Ham, extra-lean deli style	1½ oz.	2½ oz.	2½ oz.	3 oz.	4 oz.
Swiss cheese, lowfat	1 oz.	1½ oz.	1½ oz.	2 oz.	2½ oz.
Dill pickle	1	1	1	1	1
Peach, medium	½	1	1	1	1

DIRECTIONS: Grill a lightly buttered ham and cheese sandwich until golden brown on both sides. Serve with dill pickle and fresh peach.

Oriental Chicken Bowl

	A	B	C	D	E
Peanut oil	½ tbsp.	¾ tbsp.	¾ tbsp.	1 tbsp.	1⅓ tbsp.
Chicken breast, skin removed	3 oz.	4 oz.	4 oz.	5½ oz.	7 oz.
Broccoli, chopped	½ cup	1 cup	1 cup	1 cup	1 cup
Rice, cooked	½ cup	⅔ cup	⅔ cup	1 cup	1¼ cups
Soy sauce	½ tsp.	½–1 tsp.	½–1 tsp.	1 tsp.	1 tsp.

DIRECTIONS: Heat peanut oil in a skillet or wok and stir-fry chicken and broccoli. Season to taste. Serve with cooked rice and soy sauce.

MEAL PLAN PERSONAL REQUIREMENTS

Cottage Cheese, Muffin, and Fruit Plate

	A	B	C	D	E
Cottage cheese, 2% lowfat	½ cup	¾ cup	¾ cup	1 cup	1⅓ cups
Nuts (almonds, pecans, or walnuts)	1⅓ tbsp.	2⅓ tbsp.	2⅓ tbsp.	3 tbsp.	3½ tbsp.
Bran muffin, lowfat (approximately 150 calories)	½	¾	¾	1	1
Cantaloupe, medium	⅛ slice	⅛ slice	⅛ slice	¼ slice	⅓ slice
Strawberries, sliced	⅓ cup	½ cup	½ cup	½ cup	1 cup

DIRECTIONS: Sprinkle cottage cheese with sliced nuts and serve with bran muffin, cantaloupe, and strawberries.

KIDS' FAVORITE

Tuna Salad on Rye Crackers and Fruit

	A	B	C	D	E
Albacore tuna, water packed and drained	3 oz.	6 oz.	6 oz.	8 oz.	10 oz.
Sweet pickle relish	1 tsp.	2 tsp.	2 tsp.	2 tsp.	2 tsp.
Celery stalk, diced	½ stalk	½ stalk	½ stalk	½ stalk	½ stalk
Onion, diced	1 tbsp.	1 tbsp.	1 tbsp.	1 tbsp.	1 tbsp.
Mayonnaise, reduced-calorie	1¾ tbsp.	3 tbsp.	3 tbsp.	4 tbsp.	4¾ tbsp.
Rye crackers, whole grain (Wasa)	2	3⅓	3⅓	5	6
Grapes, red or green	¼ cup	⅓ cup	⅓ cup	⅓ cup	⅓ cup

DIRECTIONS: Blend tuna with pickle relish, celery, onion, and mayonnaise. Serve on rye crackers with grapes.

MEAL PLAN PERSONAL REQUIREMENTS

Boca Cheeseburger

	A	B	C	D	E
Boca Burger, fat-free	1	1½	1½	2	2½
Hamburger bun, reduced calorie	1	1	1	1	2
Cheddar cheese, full fat	½ oz.	1 oz.	1 oz.	1½ oz.	1½ oz.
Tomato slices	1	1	1	1	2
Lettuce leaves	2	2	2	2	4
Dill pickle, sliced	¼	¼	¼	½	½
Catsup	1 tsp.	1 tsp.	1 tsp.	1 tsp.	2 tsp.
Mayonnaise, full fat	1 tsp.	1 tsp.	1 tsp.	1 tsp.	1½ tsp.
Grapes	¼ cup	⅓ cup	⅓ cup	¾ cup	⅓ cup

DIRECTIONS: Heat Boca Burger patties and place on bun with cheese, tomato, lettuce, pickle, catsup, and mayonnaise. Serve with grapes. Boca Burgers are found frozen in health food and grocery stores.

Chapter Seventeen

REGULAR SNACKS

	MEAL PLAN PERSONAL REQUIREMENTS				
	A	B	C	D	E

KIDS' FAVORITE
40-30-30 Nutrition Bar

	A	B	C	D	E
40-30-30 Nutrition Bar, any flavor	1	1	1	1	2

DIRECTIONS: Have a 40-30-30 Nutrition Bar with 8–12 ounces of water.

KIDS' FAVORITE
40-30-30 Shake Mix

	A	B	C	D	E
40-30-30 shake mix, any flavor	1 packet	1 packet	1 packet	1 packet	2 packets
Water	8 ounces	8 ounces	8 ounces	8 ounces	16 ounces

DIRECTIONS: Blend 40-30-30 shake mix with water. For a thicker shake, use a blender and add ice cubes for part of the water.

KIDS' FAVORITE
Banana Walnut Smoothie

	A	B	C	D	E
Banana, medium	⅓	⅓	⅓	⅓	¾
Milk, 1% lowfat	½ cup	½ cup	½ cup	½ cup	1 cup
Granulated fructose	1 tsp.	1 tsp.	1 tsp.	1 tsp.	1½ tsp.
Pure whey protein powder	10 grams	10 grams	10 grams	10 grams	20 grams
Walnuts, chopped	1 tbsp.	1 tbsp.	1 tbsp.	1 tbsp.	2 tbsp.

DIRECTIONS: Combine all ingredients in a blender and process until smooth. For a thicker smoothie, use frozen peeled bananas.

MEAL PLAN PERSONAL REQUIREMENTS

Deli Bagel

	A	B	C	D	E
Bagel, plain, wheat, or oat bran, 3½-inch diameter	½	½	½	½	1
Cream cheese, full fat	1 tbsp.	1 tbsp.	1 tbsp.	1 tbsp.	2 tbsp.
Lean deli meat (turkey, chicken, or roast beef)	2 oz.	2 oz.	2 oz.	2 oz.	4 oz.

DIRECTIONS: Spread bagel half with cream cheese and top with sliced deli meat.

KIDS' FAVORITE

Tortilla Roll-Up

	A	B	C	D	E
Flour tortilla, 7- to 8-inch diameter	1	1	1	1	2
Mayonnaise, full fat	1 tsp.	1 tsp.	1 tsp.	1 tsp.	2 tsp.
Lean deli meat (turkey, chicken, or roast beef)	2½ oz.	2½ oz.	2½ oz.	2½ oz.	5 oz.

DIRECTIONS: Spread flour tortilla with mayonnaise. Top with deli meat and roll up.

Wine and Cheese

	A	B	C	D	E
Cheese, 50% reduced fat, any kind	2 oz.	2 oz.	2 oz.	2 oz.	4 oz.
Wine, red or white	4 oz.	4 oz.	4 oz.	4 oz.	6 oz.
Almonds, sliced	2 tsp.	2 tsp.	2 tsp.	2 tsp.	1 tbsp.

DIRECTIONS: Have a glass of wine with lowfat cheese and almonds.

Crab Cocktail

	A	B	C	D	E
Crab or lobster meat, cooked	2 oz.	2 oz.	2 oz.	2 oz.	3½ oz.
Shredded lettuce	½ cup	½ cup	½ cup	½ cup	¾ cup
Cocktail sauce, prepared	⅓ cup	⅓ cup	⅓ cup	⅓ cup	⅔ cup
Nuts (almonds, pecans, or walnuts), chopped	1⅓ tbsp.	1⅓ tbsp.	1⅓ tbsp.	1⅓ tbsp.	2⅓ tbsp.

DIRECTIONS: Place chilled crab or lobster meat in a lettuce-lined cup with cocktail sauce. Serve with nuts.

	MEAL PLAN PERSONAL REQUIREMENTS				
	A	**B**	**C**	**D**	**E**
Shrimp Cocktail					
Shrimp, large, cooked	2 oz.	2 oz.	2 oz.	2 oz.	3½ oz.
Shredded lettuce	½ cup	½ cup	½ cup	½ cup	¾ cup
Cocktail sauce, prepared	⅓ cup	⅓ cup	⅓ cup	⅓ cup	⅔ cup
Nuts (almonds, pecans, or walnuts), chopped	1½ tbsp.	1½ tbsp.	1½ tbsp.	1½ tbsp.	2⅓ tbsp.

DIRECTIONS: Shell and devein freshly cooked shrimp. Chill and serve in a lettuce-lined cup with cocktail sauce. Serve with nuts.

KIDS' FAVORITE
Chicken Quesadilla

	A	B	C	D	E
Flour tortilla, 7- to 8-inch diameter	1	1	1	1	2
Cooked chicken, diced	1½ oz.	1½ oz.	1½ oz.	1½ oz.	3 oz.
Jack or Cheddar cheese, full fat, shredded	2 tbsp.	2 tbsp.	2 tbsp.	2 tbsp.	3 tbsp.
Salsa	2 tbsp.	2 tbsp.	2 tbsp.	2 tbsp.	4 tbsp.

DIRECTIONS: Heat tortilla in a nonstick pan, top with cooked chicken and grated cheese, and cook until melted. Fold and serve topped with salsa.

KIDS' FAVORITE
Cheese Quesadilla

	A	B	C	D	E
Flour tortilla, 7- to 8-inch diameter	1	1	1	1	2
Jack or Cheddar cheese, reduced fat, grated	½ cup	½ cup	½ cup	½ cup	1 cup
Diced green chili peppers, mild or hot	1 tbsp.	1 tbsp.	1 tbsp.	1 tbsp.	1 tbsp.
Black olives, large	3	3	3	3	2

DIRECTIONS: Heat tortilla in a nonstick skillet and sprinkle with grated cheese until melted. Add chilies and sliced olives; fold and serve.

MEAL PLAN PERSONAL REQUIREMENTS

	A	B	C	D	E
Chips and Dip					
Cottage cheese, 2% lowfat	½ cup	½ cup	½ cup	½ cup	¾ cup
Salsa	3 tbsp.	3 tbsp.	3 tbsp.	3 tbsp.	5 tbsp.
Corn tortilla chips, white or yellow	¾ oz.	¾ oz.	¾ oz.	¾ oz.	1⅓ oz.

DIRECTIONS: Mix cottage cheese and salsa. Serve as a dip with chips.

	A	B	C	D	E
California Rolls (Sushi)					
California rolls, approximately 2-inch diameter	3	3	3	3	6

DIRECTIONS: Look for premade California rolls that contain tuna or salmon, cucumber, and cream cheese rolled in rice.

Chapter Eighteen

REGULAR DINNERS

MEAL PLAN PERSONAL REQUIREMENTS

KIDS' FAVORITE

Beef Kabobs with Fried Rice

	A	B	C	D	E
Top loin beef, extra lean, cubed	3 oz.	3½ oz.	4½ oz.	4½ oz.	5½ oz.
Teriyaki marinade, bottled	1 tbsp.	1 tbsp.	2 tbsp.	2 tbsp.	2 tbsp.
Green or red bell pepper, medium, cubed	⅓	⅓	½	½	½
Sweet onion, cubed	¼	¼	½	½	½
Cherry tomatoes	4	4	6	6	6
FRIED RICE:					
Brown and wild rice blend	3 tbsp.	¼ cup	¼ cup	¼ cup	⅓ cup
Beef broth, canned	½ cup	½ cup	½ cup	½ cup	⅔ cup
Olive oil	1½ tsp.	1½ tsp.	2 tsp.	2 tsp.	2 tsp.
Carrots, diced	2 tbsp.	3 tbsp.	¼ cup	¼ cup	¼ cup
Celery, diced	2 tbsp.	3 tbsp.	¼ cup	¼ cup	¼ cup

FRIED RICE RECIPE: Cook rice in beef broth. In a frying pan, heat oil and sauté carrots and celery until tender. Add cooked rice and toss.

DIRECTIONS: Marinate beef cubes in teriyaki marinade for 20 to 30 minutes. On several skewers, alternate marinated beef cubes, bell pepper, onion, and tomatoes. Grill or broil and serve with fried rice.

MEAL PLAN PERSONAL REQUIREMENTS

Macaroni and Cheese with Chicken Dinner

	A	B	C	D	E
Macaroni and Cheese (see recipe)	¾ cup	1 cup	1¼ cups	1¼ cups	1½ cups
Chicken breast (cooked amount)	2½ oz.	2½ oz.	3 oz.	3 oz.	4 oz.
Green beans, fresh or canned	¾ cup	1 cup	1 cup	1 cup	1½ cups
Peach, fresh, medium (or ½ cup canned, drained)	1	1	1	1	1

MACARONI AND CHEESE

3 cups macaroni, cooked, elbow
3 tablespoons olive oil
2 tablespoons flour
½ teaspoon salt
⅛ teaspoon pepper
2 cups milk, 1% lowfat
8 ounces cheddar cheese, lowfat

MACARONI AND CHEESE DIRECTIONS: Preheat oven to 350°F. In a saucepan, heat oil and blend in flour, salt, and pepper. Add milk and stir until thick and bubbly. Add cheese chunks until melted. Add cooked macaroni and mix thoroughly. Place in a casserole dish and bake for 35 minutes or until heated through and lightly browned.

DIRECTIONS: Serve Macaroni and Cheese with chicken, green beans, and peach.

Thai Chicken Pizza

	A	B	C	D	E
Flour tortilla, 7- to 8-inch diameter	1½	1¾	2	2	2½
Peanut sauce	2 tbsp.	2 tbsp.	2⅓ tbsp.	2⅓ tbsp.	3 tbsp.
Cooked chicken breast	3 oz.	3½ oz.	4 oz.	4 oz.	5 oz.
Carrots, shredded	1⅓ tbsp.	1⅓ tbsp.	1½ tbsp.	1½ tbsp.	2½ tbsp.
Bean sprouts, fresh	⅓ cup	⅓ cup	⅓ cup	⅓ cup	½ cup
Mixed salad greens	2 cups	2 cups	2 cups	2 cups	2 cups
Salad dressing, fat-free, any kind	1 tbsp.	1 tbsp.	1 tbsp.	1 tbsp.	1 tbsp.

DIRECTIONS: Preheat oven to 400°F. Place tortillas on a baking sheet and bake until crisp. Spread with peanut sauce and top with cooked chicken and shredded carrots. Return to oven for 10 minutes until hot. Remove and top with bean sprouts. Serve with a salad and dressing.

	MEAL PLAN PERSONAL REQUIREMENTS				
	A	B	C	D	E

KIDS' FAVORITE

BBQ Chicken Pizza

	A	B	C	D	E
Flour tortillas, 7- to 8-inch diameter	1½	1¾	2	2	2½
Barbecue sauce, bottled	1½ tbsp.	2 tbsp.	2 tbsp.	2 tbsp.	2½ tbsp.
Cooked chicken breast, cubed	2½ oz.	3 oz.	4 oz.	4 oz.	4½ oz.
Red onion, sliced thin	1½ slices	1¾ slices	2 slices	2 slices	2½ slices
Cilantro, chopped	1 tsp.	1 tsp.	2 tsp.	2 tsp.	2 tsp.
Gouda cheese, grated	¼ cup	¼ cup	⅓ cup	⅓ cup	½ cup
Mixed salad greens	2 cups	2 cups	2 cups	2 cups	2 cups
Salad dressing, fat-free, any kind	1 tbsp.	1 tbsp.	1 tbsp.	1 tbsp.	1 tbsp.

DIRECTIONS: Preheat oven to 400°F. Place tortillas on a baking sheet and bake until crisp. Spread with barbecue sauce and top with cooked chicken, onions, cilantro, and cheese. Return to oven for 10 to 15 minutes until cheese melts and begins to brown. Serve with a salad and dressing.

Pesto Chicken Pizza

	A	B	C	D	E
Flour tortillas, 7- to 8-inch diameter	2	2¼	2½	2½	3
Pesto sauce	1 tbsp.	1⅓ tbsp.	2 tbsp.	2 tbsp.	2 tbsp.
Cooked chicken breast, cubed	3½ oz.	3½ oz.	4 oz.	4 oz.	5½ oz.
Green onion, chopped	2 tbsp.	2 tbsp.	2½ tbsp.	2½ tbsp.	3 tbsp.
Mixed salad greens	1½ cups	1½ cups	1½ cups	1½ cups	1½ cups
Salad dressing, fat-free, any kind	1 tbsp.	1 tbsp.	1 tbsp.	1 tbsp.	1 tbsp.

DIRECTIONS: Preheat oven to 400°F. Place tortillas on a baking sheet and bake until crisp. Spread with pesto sauce and top with cooked chicken and green onions. Return to oven for 10 to 15 minutes until hot. Serve with a salad and dressing.

	MEAL PLAN PERSONAL REQUIREMENTS				
	A	B	C	D	E

KIDS' FAVORITE

Gene's Favorite Pizza

	A	B	C	D	E
Flour tortillas, 7- to 8-inch diameter	1½	1¾	2	2	2½
Pizza sauce	3 tbsp.	¼ cup	¼ cup	¼ cup	⅓ cup
Turkey sausage, mild to hot, cooked	2 oz.	2 oz.	2 oz.	2 oz.	3 oz.
Mushroom slices	¼ cup	¼ cup	⅓ cup	⅓ cup	⅓ cup
Onion, chopped	1 tbsp.	1½ tbsp.	2 tbsp.	2 tbsp.	2½ tbsp.
Black olives, large	3	3	6	6	6
Mozzarella cheese, part skim, shredded	⅓ cup	½ cup	½ cup	½ cup	⅔ cup
Parmesan cheese, grated	1½ tbsp.	1½ tbsp.	2 tbsp.	2 tbsp.	2 tbsp.
Mixed salad greens	1½ cups	1½ cups	1½ cups	1½ cups	1½ cups
Salad dressing, fat-free, any kind	1 tbsp.	1 tbsp.	1 tbsp.	1 tbsp.	1 tbsp.

DIRECTIONS: Preheat oven to 400°F. Place tortillas on a baking sheet and bake until crisp. Spread with pizza sauce and top with cooked sausage, mushrooms, onions, black olives, and mozzarella and Parmesan cheeses. Return to oven for 10 to 15 minutes until cheese melts and begins to brown. Serve with a salad and dressing.

KIDS' FAVORITE

Hawaiian Pizza

	A	B	C	D	E
Flour tortillas, 7- to 8-inch diameter	1½	1¾	2	2	2½
Pizza sauce	1½ tbsp.	1¾ tbsp.	2 tbsp.	2 tbsp.	2½ tbsp.
Canadian bacon, diced	4 oz.	4 oz.	4½ oz.	4½ oz.	5½ oz.
Pineapple rings, canned, drained	1 ring	1 ring	1 ring	1 ring	1½ rings
Mozzarella cheese, shredded	2 tbsp.	2 tbsp.	3 tbsp.	3 tbsp.	¼ cup
Mixed salad greens	2 cups	2 cups	2 cups	2 cups	2 cups
Salad dressing, fat-free, any kind	1 tbsp.	1 tbsp.	1 tbsp.	1 tbsp.	1 tbsp.

DIRECTIONS: Preheat oven to 400°F. Place tortillas on a baking sheet and bake until crisp. Spread tortilla with pizza sauce and top with diced Canadian bacon, pineapple chunks, and cheese. Return to oven for 10 to 15 minutes until cheese melts and begins to brown. Serve with a salad and dressing.

	MEAL PLAN PERSONAL REQUIREMENTS				
	A	**B**	**C**	**D**	**E**

KIDS' FAVORITE

Cheese Pizza

	A	B	C	D	E
Flour tortillas, 7- to 8-inch diameter	1⅔	2	2	2	2½
Pizza sauce	3 tbsp.	3 tbsp.	4 tbsp.	4 tbsp.	6 tbsp.
Mozzarella cheese, part skim, shredded	½ cup	½ cup	½ cup	½ cup	⅔ cup
Mozzarella cheese, nonfat, shredded	⅓ cup	⅓ cup	½ cup	½ cup	⅔ cup

DIRECTIONS: Preheat oven to 400°F. Place tortillas on a baking sheet and bake until crisp. Spread tortilla with pizza sauce and top with cheese. Return to oven for 10 to 15 minutes until cheese melts and begins to brown.

KIDS' FAVORITE

Chicken Cheese Crisp (Mexican Pizza)

	A	B	C	D	E
Flour tortillas, 7- to 8-inch diameter	2	2	2½	2½	3
Jalapeño cheese, shredded	2½ tbsp.	2½ tbsp.	3 tbsp.	3 tbsp.	4 tbsp.
Cheddar cheese, 50% reduced fat, shredded	2 tbsp.	2 tbsp.	2½ tbsp.	2½ tbsp.	3 tbsp.
Green chiles, canned or fresh, diced	2 tbsp.	2 tbsp.	2½ tbsp.	2½ tbsp.	3 tbsp.
Cooked chicken breast, cubed	2½ oz.	3 oz.	3½ oz.	3½ oz.	4½ oz.
Black olives, large	4	6	6	6	6

DIRECTIONS: Preheat oven to 400°F. Place tortillas on a baking sheet, spray lightly with olive oil spray, and bake until crisp. Top tortilla with jalapeño and cheddar cheese, chilies, chicken, and sliced olives. Return to oven for 10 to 15 minutes until cheese melts and begins to brown.

	MEAL PLAN PERSONAL REQUIREMENTS				
	A	**B**	**C**	**D**	**E**

KIDS' FAVORITE/ *Family Style*

Sloppy Joes in Pita Pocket

	A	B	C	D	E
Sloppy Joe mixture (recipe below)	1 cup	1½ cups	2 cups	2 cups	2½ cups
Pita bread, wheat or white, 6½″ size	1	1½	2	2	2½
Peaches, fresh sliced or canned in water, drained	¾ cup	¾ cup	1 cup	1 cup	1½ cup

SLOPPY JOES

2 tablespoons olive oil

½ cup minced onion

½ cup chopped celery

½ cup chopped green pepper

1 garlic clove, minced

1 pound ground turkey breast or extra-lean ground sirloin

½ cup chopped mushrooms

¼ cup bottled chili sauce

½ cup catsup

1 teaspoon Worcestershire sauce

½ cup water

SLOPPY JOE DIRECTIONS: Heat oil in a skillet and sauté onions, celery, green pepper, and garlic until soft and just beginning to brown. Add ground meat and brown. Add mushrooms, chili sauce, catsup, Worcestershire sauce, and water. Simmer for 15 to 20 minutes uncovered.

DIRECTIONS: Serve Sloppy Joes in pita bread halves with peaches on the side.

MEAL PLAN PERSONAL REQUIREMENTS

Soft Fish Tacos

	A	B	C	D	E
White fish fillet, cod, raw	4½ oz.	5 oz.	6 oz.	6 oz.	8 oz.
Olive oil	¼ tsp.	½ tsp.	½ tsp.	½ tsp.	1¼ tsp.
Sour cream, lowfat	¼ cup	¼ cup	⅓ cup	⅓ cup	⅓ cup
Mexican seasonings	½ tsp.	½ tsp.	⅔ tsp.	⅔ tsp.	⅔ tsp.
Corn tortillas, 5-inch diameter	2	3	3	3	4
Cabbage, shredded	⅓ cup	⅓ cup	½ cup	½ cup	⅔ cup
Salsa	3 tbsp.	3 tbsp.	3 tbsp.	3 tbsp.	¼ cup
Avocado, medium	¼	¼	¼	¼	⅓

DIRECTIONS: Heat olive oil in a nonstick pan and cook fish until done. Blend sour cream with Mexican seasonings. Warm corn tortillas and fill with fish, sour cream mixture, cabbage, salsa, and avocado slices. Fold in half and serve.

KIDS' FAVORITE

Spaghetti and Meatballs

	A	B	C	D	E
Extra-lean ground sirloin	3 oz.	3½ oz.	4 oz.	4 oz.	5 oz.
Egg, white only	1	1	1	1	1
Italian bread crumbs	2 tsp.	1 tbsp.	1½ tbsp.	1½ tbsp.	1½ tbsp.
Italian seasonings	1 tsp.	1 tsp.	1 tsp.	1 tsp.	1½ tsp.
Spaghetti sauce, bottled, canned, or homemade	½ cup	½ cup	½ cup	½ cup	¾ cup
Spaghetti, cooked	½ cup	⅔ cup	¾ cup	¾ cup	1 cup
Parmesan cheese, grated	2 tsp.	1 tbsp.	1 tbsp.	1 tbsp.	2 tbsp.
Mixed salad greens	2 cups	2 cups	2 cups	2 cups	2 cups
Italian salad dressing (Newman's Own)	1½ tbsp.	1½ tbsp.	2 tbsp.	2 tbsp.	2 tbsp.

DIRECTIONS: Mix ground sirloin with egg white, bread crumbs, and Italian seasonings. Form small meatballs and brown slowly in a nonstick pan. Add spaghetti sauce and simmer for 20 minutes. Pour over cooked pasta sprinkled with Parmesan cheese. Serve with a salad and dressing.

MEAL PLAN PERSONAL REQUIREMENTS

	A	B	C	D	E

KIDS' FAVORITE/ *Family Style*

Lasagna

	A	B	C	D	E
Lasagna (recipe below)	1¼ slices	1½ slices	1¾ slices	1¾ slices	2 slices
Mixed salad greens	1½ cups	1½ cups	2 cups	2 cups	2 cups
Olive oil and vinegar salad dressing (Newman's Own)	2 tsp.	2 tsp.	1 tbsp.	1 tbsp.	1 tbsp.

LASAGNA

8 ounces lasagna noodles

½ pound ground sirloin, lean

1 cup ricotta cheese

1 cup nonfat cottage cheese

2 tablespoons fresh parsley

1 egg

1 egg white

1 teaspoon salt

½ teaspoon pepper

3 cups pasta sauce

1¼ cups part-skim mozzarella cheese, grated

3 tablespoons Parmesan cheese

RECIPE DIRECTIONS: Preheat oven to 375°F. Cook lasagna noodles according to package directions; drain and cool. Brown ground sirloin and drain any excess fat. In a large bowl, combine ricotta and cottage cheese, parsley, egg and egg white, salt, and pepper. Lightly coat a 9 × 13–inch baking pan with olive oil spray. Spread ½ cup pasta sauce in the bottom of pan. Line the pan with half of the lasagna noodles and spread with half of the cheese mixture. Sprinkle evenly with cooked ground sirloin. Top with half of the remaining pasta sauce. Layer the remaining lasagna noodles, cheese mixture, and sauce. Top with grated mozzarella cheese and Parmesan cheese. Bake in oven for 30 to 40 minutes until hot, bubbly, and brown. Cut in 8 equal slices.

DIRECTIONS: Serve Lasagna with salad and dressing.

MEAL PLAN PERSONAL REQUIREMENTS

KIDS' FAVORITE
Shredded Chicken Burritos

	A	B	C	D	E
Flour tortilla, 7- to 8-inch diameter	1½	1¾	2	2	2½
Sour cream, full fat	2 tbsp.	2⅓ tbsp.	2¾ tbsp.	2¾ tbsp.	3 tbsp.
Refried beans, canned	1½ tbsp.	2 tbsp.	2 tbsp.	2 tbsp.	2½ tbsp.
Shredded Chicken (recipe below)	⅔ cup	⅔ cup	¾ cup	¾ cup	1 cup
Lettuce, shredded	¼ cup	¼ cup	⅓ cup	⅓ cup	⅓ cup
Tomato, chopped	¼ cup	¼ cup	⅓ cup	⅓ cup	⅓ cup
Salsa	3 tbsp.	3 tbsp.	3 tbsp.	3 tbsp.	3 tbsp.

SHREDDED CHICKEN

2 pounds chicken, breast meat only
¼ cup water
3 tablespoons red wine vinegar
1½ cups chicken broth
2 tablespoons chili powder
1 teaspoon ground cumin

SHREDDED CHICKEN DIRECTIONS: Place chicken breasts in a 5- to 6-quart pot with water and cook over medium heat for 30 minutes. Uncover and cook until liquid evaporates and chicken begins to brown. In a bowl, blend vinegar, chicken broth, chili powder, and cumin. Add to meat and continue cooking over medium heat until chicken is very tender and pulls apart easily (about 1 hour). Let chicken cool; shred it with two forks. Mix with remaining juices.

DIRECTIONS: Place sour cream, refried beans, and shredded chicken mixture on warmed flour tortilla. Top with lettuce, tomato, and salsa. Fold burrito style.

MEAL PLAN PERSONAL REQUIREMENTS				
A	B	C	D	E

Family Style

Hoagie Sandwich

	A	B	C	D	E
Hoagie Sandwich	1½ slices	1¾ slices	2 slices	2 slices	2⅓ slices
Dill pickle	½	¾	1	1	1¾

HOAGIE SANDWICH RECIPE:

1 whole French bread loaf, 14 to
    15 inches long, white or whole wheat
1 pound deli-style turkey breast
¼ pound deli-style lowfat Swiss cheese
2 cups shredded lettuce
2 whole tomatoes, thinly sliced
½ sweet onion, thinly sliced
½ green bell pepper, thinly sliced
¾ avocado, mashed
2 tablespoons mustard
2 tablespoons Italian salad dressing, full fat

HOAGIE SANDWICH DIRECTIONS: Slice French bread in half horizontally and hollow out both halves by discarding the soft inside bread. Fill one half with turkey and cheese slices. Top with shredded lettuce and thinly sliced tomato, onion, and green pepper. Spread the avocado evenly in other half. Spread with mustard and drizzle with Italian dressing. Place both halves together and slice into 8 even portions to serve.

DIRECTIONS: Serve Hoagie Sandwich with dill pickle.

Grilled Salmon Dinner

	MEAL PLAN PERSONAL REQUIREMENTS				
	A	B	C	D	E
Salmon steak or fillet	4 oz.	5 oz.	6 oz.	6 oz.	7 oz.
Red potatoes, 2½-inch diameter, cooked	1⅓	1½	2	2	2½
Asparagus spears, steamed	10	10	10	10	12
Mixed salad greens	2 cups	2 cups	2 cups	2 cups	2½ cups
Italian salad dressing, full fat	2 tbsp.	2 tbsp.	2 tbsp.	2 tbsp.	2½ tbsp.

DIRECTIONS: Broil or grill salmon steak. Season with salt, pepper, garlic, and lemon juice to taste. Serve with cooked red potatoes, steamed asparagus, and a mixed green salad with dressing.

KIDS' FAVORITE / Family Style

Taco Soup Dinner

	A	B	C	D	E
Taco Soup (recipe below)	1¾ cup	2 cups	2½ cups	2½ cups	3¼ cups
Sour cream, lowfat	2 tbsp.	2 tbsp.	3 tbsp.	3 tbsp.	3½ tbsp.
Cheddar cheese, full fat, shredded	1 tbsp.	1 tbsp.	2 tbsp.	2 tbsp.	3 tbsp.
Corn taco shell, small size, crumbled	1	1	2	2	3

TACO SOUP

1½ pounds extra-lean ground sirloin

1 tablespoon olive oil

1 cup diced onion

1 clove garlic, minced

28-ounce can diced tomatoes, with juice

15-ounce can tomato sauce

15¼-ounce can black beans, with juice

8¾-ounce can corn, with juice

1-ounce package of taco seasoning mix

TACO SOUP DIRECTIONS: In a medium heavy pot, heat oil. Add the ground sirloin and brown. Add onion and garlic and cook for 5 minutes. Add canned tomatoes, tomato sauce, beans, corn, and taco seasoning mix. Cook 30 minutes longer.

DIRECTIONS: In a bowl, serve taco soup topped with sour cream, cheese, and crumbled taco shell.

MEAL PLAN PERSONAL REQUIREMENTS

KIDS' FAVORITE / Family Style

Old-Fashioned Beef Stew

	A	B	C	D	E
Beef Stew (recipe below)	1¾ cups	2 cups	2⅓ cups	2⅓ cups	2¾ cups
Mixed salad greens	2 cups	2 cups	2 cups	2 cups	2½ cups
Italian salad dressing, full fat	2 tsp.	2 tsp.	1 tbsp.	1 tbsp.	1½ tbsp.
Peaches, fresh or canned in water, drained	1 cup	1 cup	1½ cups	1½ cups	1¾ cups

BEEF STEW

1 tablespoon olive oil

1½ pounds lean stew beef cubes, trimmed of visible fat

2⅓ cups water, divided

1 tablespoon Worcestershire sauce

1 clove garlic, minced

½ cup onion, chopped

2 bay leaves

1 tablespoon salt

1 teaspoon granulated fructose

½ teaspoon paprika

½ teaspoon black pepper

¼ teaspoon allspice

3 cups sliced carrots

3 cups cubed red potatoes

2½ cups pearl onions

3 tablespoons flour

RECIPE DIRECTIONS: In a heavy pan, heat olive oil and brown beef cubes. Add 2 cups of water, Worcestershire sauce, garlic, onion, bay leaves, salt, fructose, paprika, pepper, and allspice. Cover and simmer for 1½ hours, stirring occasionally to prevent sticking. Remove bay leaves. Add carrots, potatoes, and onions; cover and cook 30 minutes longer until vegetables are tender. In a small cup, whisk ⅓ cup water and flour and stir into the hot stew to thicken and serve.

DIRECTIONS: Serve Old-Fashioned Beef Stew with a green salad with salad dressing and peaches.

	MEAL PLAN PERSONAL REQUIREMENTS				
	A	**B**	**C**	**D**	**E**

Tuna Pasta Caesar Salad

	A	B	C	D	E
Romaine lettuce, washed and torn	⅓ head	½ head	½ head	½ head	½ head
Cheese-filled tortellini, cooked	⅔ cup	¾ cup	1 cup	1 cup	1½ cups
Albacore tuna, water-packed, canned, drained	3 oz.	3 oz.	3½ oz.	3½ oz.	4 oz.
Caesar Salad Dressing (recipe below)	1⅔ tbsp.	1⅔ tbsp.	2⅓ tbsp.	2⅓ tbsp.	2⅔ tbsp.
Croutons, plain or seasoned	⅓ cup	⅓ cup	⅓ cup	⅓ cup	⅓ cup
Parmesan cheese, grated	1 tbsp.	1⅓ tbsp.	1½ tbsp.	1½ tbsp.	1½ tbsp.

CAESAR SALAD DRESSING

3 tablespoons olive oil

2 tablespoons red wine vinegar

1 tablespoon lemon juice, fresh or
   bottled

1 teaspoon Worcestershire sauce

1 small clove garlic, pressed, or
   ½ teaspoon garlic powder

1 teaspoon anchovy paste (from tube)

⅛ teaspoon salt

⅛ teaspoon pepper

½ teaspoon dry mustard

CAESAR SALAD DRESSING DIRECTIONS: Place all ingredients in a small jar and shake well.

DIRECTIONS: Add cooked tuna and tortellini to romaine lettuce. Toss with Caesar Salad Dressing and top with croutons and grated Parmesan cheese.

KIDS' FAVORITE

Summertime Barbecued Chicken Dinner

	MEAL PLAN PERSONAL REQUIREMENTS				
	A	B	C	D	E
Chicken breast, skinless	3½ oz.	4 oz.	5 oz.	5 oz.	6 oz.
Barbecue sauce, bottled	1½ tbsp.	2 tbsp.	2 tbsp.	2 tbsp.	2 tbsp.
Corn on the cob, medium ear	½ ear	½ ear	1 ear	1 ear	1½ ears
Whipped butter	½ tsp.	½ tsp.	1 tsp.	1 tsp.	1½ tsp.
Green beans, fresh or canned	1¼ cups	1½ cups	1½ cups	1½ cups	2 cups
Almonds, sliced	2 tbsp.	2 tbsp.	2 tbsp.	2 tbsp.	2 tbsp.
Dill pickle	½	1 whole	1 whole	1 whole	1 whole
Strawberries, fresh sliced	1½ cups	1½ cups	1½ cups	1½ cups	1½ cups

DIRECTIONS: Grill chicken breast and baste with barbecue sauce. Serve with buttered corn on the cob. Salt and pepper to taste. Serve with green beans with sliced almonds, a pickle, and strawberries for dessert.

Chapter Nineteen

REGULAR DESSERTS

The following dessert recipes are easy to prepare, have been kitchen tested, and were all designed with the 40-30-30 ratio in mind. These recipes include a variety of high and low glycemic carbohydrates. For that reason, we classify them as Regular Formula Desserts; these should be used as a part of your Formula for Life maintenance program. You can eat a dessert for an occasional afternoon snack, as a snack before bed, or for special holiday events. Of course, you still need to be aware of the total calories you consume each day. The 40-30-30 Formula dessert recipes take the guesswork out of making and eating desserts.

All of the dessert recipes contain 30% of calories from high quality protein sources. Each recipe has been fortified with pure whey protein powder. Pure whey protein powder is an excellent source of quality protein, has little or no taste, mixes instantly, and can be used in cooking and baking. It is derived from dairy, but is lactose free. Use a whey protein powder that is 90% pure, contains no sweeteners or flavors, and has little if any fat or carbohydrate.

Look for a pure whey protein powder with the following nutritional profile:

PURE WHEY PROTEIN POWDER

Serving size:	1 scoop (22.2 gram size)
Calories:	80
Carbohydrate	0 grams
Protein	20 grams
Fat	0 grams

If you have trouble finding a source of pure whey protein powder, call Craig Nutraceuticals at 800-293-1683.

KIDS' FAVORITE
PUMPKIN MOUSSE CHEESECAKE

If you enjoy pumpkin pie, you'll love this cheesecake.
Served warm or cold, it's a lot like pumpkin pie, only richer.

8	ounces Philadelphia Brand Fat Free Cream Cheese
4	ounces Philadelphia Brand ⅓ Less Fat Cream Cheese
⅛	cup granulated fructose
¼	cup brown sugar
2	large eggs
2	tablespoons lowfat sour cream
1	cup canned pumpkin
¼	teaspoon salt
½	teaspoon vanilla
¼	teaspoon ground ginger
½	teaspoon ground cinnamon
⅛	teaspoon ground cloves
30	grams of pure whey protein powder
8	tablespoons of whipped cream

Preheat oven to 325°F. Lightly grease and flour an 8-inch round cake pan. In a large bowl, blend cream cheese, fructose, and brown sugar. Mix in eggs, sour cream, pumpkin, salt, vanilla, and spices. Blend in pure whey protein powder. Pour the mixture into the prepared pan.

Bake the cake on the center rack for 35 minutes or until just set in the middle. Serve warm or chilled with whipped cream. Cake can be stored covered with plastic wrap in the refrigerator for up to 8 days, or frozen. Makes 8 servings.

Per serving: 150 calories; Grams = C-15g, P-11g, F-5g

ORANGE WALNUT
BUNDT CAKE

This delicious cake is extra rich and moist. The flavors and textures
of the nuts, orange, and cheese complement each other perfectly.

1	cup flour
95	grams of pure whey protein powder
2	teaspoons baking powder
½	teaspoon salt
¼	cup butter
2	(8-ounce) blocks Philadelphia Brand Fat Free Cream Cheese
1	teaspoon grated orange peel
¾	cup granulated fructose
5	large egg whites
½	cup walnuts
¼	cup milk, divided
2	tablespoons sifted powdered sugar
⅛	teaspoon orange extract (or fresh orange juice)
1	teaspoon egg white
1	tablespoon finely chopped walnuts

Preheat oven to 300°F. Thoroughly grease and flour a 3-quart bundt pan.
Sift together flour, whey protein powder, baking powder, and salt. Set aside.

In a large mixing bowl, cream butter. Add cream cheese, orange peel, and fructose, and mix well. Add egg whites one at a time until well blended.

Add half of the flour mixture and half of the milk to the batter and mix well. Add the remaining flour mixture and milk and blend well. Stir in the walnuts.

Pour the batter into the prepared bundt pan and bake for 1 hour and 15 minutes or until a knife inserted into the middle of the cake comes out clean. Oven temperatures may vary. *Do not overbake* or cake will become dry.

Remove the cake from pan and cool on a wire rack.

Blend powdered sugar, orange extract, and 1 teaspoon egg white. Drizzle over the top of the cake and sprinkle with 1 tablespoon finely chopped walnuts. Makes 24 servings.

Per serving: 115 calories; Grams = C-12g, P-9g, F-4g

KIDS' FAVORITE
OATMEAL COCONUT BALLS

◆

These healthy, fiber-rich cookies taste more like candy and are ready to serve in less than 10 minutes. Oatmeal, cocoa, coconut, and peanut butter blend to make these little nuggets irresistible.

2 tablespoons natural peanut butter (creamy or chunky)

¼ cup uncooked oatmeal

½ cup water

2½ tablespoons granulated fructose

55 grams of pure whey protein powder

3 tablespoons unsweetened cocoa powder

4 tablespoons flaked coconut

Blend all ingredients in a quart-size, microwave-safe glass bowl.

Microwave on High for 1 minute. Batter will be cooked around the edge and runny in the center. Stir mixture well with a fork. Microwaves can vary. If after stirring the batter it is still runny, return it to the microwave for 15 to 30 seconds. Batter should be moist but not runny.

Drop cookies from a teaspoon onto wax paper and form into balls. Mixture will be hot to handle. As cookies begin to set, place on wire rack to continue cooling. Store in an airtight container in the refrigerator. Makes about 18 cookies.

Per cookie: 57 calories; Grams = C-6g, P-4g, F-1.8g

KIDS' FAVORITE
CHOCOLATE PEANUT BUTTER SHAKE

If you love frozen yogurt, you'll love this frozen milk shake.
We blended frozen yogurt with protein powder and peanut butter,
and presto! A creamy, delicious, 40-30-30 Formula milk shake.

¾ cup lowfat vanilla frozen yogurt

⅓ cup nonfat milk

2 teaspoons natural peanut butter

1 tablespoon unsweetened cocoa powder

15 grams of pure whey protein powder

Combine frozen yogurt, milk, and peanut butter in a blender and process
    until smooth.

Add cocoa powder and whey protein powder and blend.

Pour into two small glasses and serve at once. Makes two servings.

Per serving: 170 calories; Grams = C-17.5g, P-13g, F-5.25g

KIDS' FAVORITE
FROZEN CHOCOLATE PIE

*This dark, rich, frozen ice cream pie is perfect for
summertime birthdays. Top it with candles and make
your special occasion a cool 40-30-30 Formula one.*

4	sheets honey or chocolate graham crackers (5 inches × 2½ inches per sheet)
15	grams of pure whey protein powder
2	tablespoons butter, melted
1	tablespoon water
2	cups lowfat frozen vanilla yogurt or lowfat ice cream
½	cup nonfat milk
2	tablespoons unsweetened cocoa powder
70	grams of pure whey protein powder

Place the graham crackers in a plastic baggie and crush them into fine
crumbs. Place crumbs in a bowl and blend in 15 grams of whey protein powder. Add melted butter and water and stir with a fork until
well blended. Pour crumbs into an 8-inch pie pan and press to form
pie shell.

Combine frozen yogurt and nonfat milk in a blender and process until
smooth. Blend in cocoa powder and whey protein powder. Pour

into pie shell and refreeze immediately for 2 hours or overnight. If frozen overnight, let pie soften slightly before slicing. Makes 8 servings.

Per serving: 165 calories; Grams = C-16.5g, P-13g, F-5.5g

ALMOND BISCOTTI

You don't have to be Italian to love these crunchy little cookies!
They're great to dunk in a cup of decaffeinated coffee or tea,
and fit the bill as the perfect little after-dinner treat.

⅓ cup almonds

3 tablespoons butter

½ cup granulated fructose

1 tablespoon grated orange peel

2 medium egg whites

1 teaspoon vanilla

100 grams of pure whey protein powder

¾ cup flour

2½ teaspoons baking powder

½ teaspoon salt

¼ teaspoon ground cinnamon

⅛ teaspoon ground cloves

⅛ teaspoon ground nutmeg

Preheat oven to 350°F. Lightly butter a large baking sheet.

Place almonds in a small pan and roast in oven, shaking often until golden, about 10 minutes; let cool.

In a large bowl, beat together butter, fructose, and orange peel. Add egg whites and vanilla and mix well.

Combine whey protein powder, flour, baking powder, salt, spices, and toasted almonds. Add to butter mixture and blend thoroughly. Dough will be rather dry.

Place dough on a floured board to prevent sticking. Divide into two equal pieces and pat each into an evenly thick rectangle that measures 12 inches × 3½ inches. Carefully transfer dough rectangles to the baking sheet. Bake for 15 minutes, using a timer.

Remove biscotti from oven and, using a large knife, cut each rectangle crosswise into 18 even slices. Tip each slice onto a cut side.

Reduce oven heat to 300°F. Return sliced cookies to oven and continue baking until golden brown, about 30 minutes; turn cookies over once while baking. Cool on racks. Store in airtight tins or freeze. Makes 36 cookies.

Per cookie: 50 calories; Grams = C-5g, P-4, F-1.75

KIDS' FAVORITE
MICROWAVE FUDGE BROWNIE

If you like moist, gooey chocolate brownies, prepare to be in chocolate heaven when you try these rich, fudge treats. These can be made in a snap, since the "baking" time is only a few minutes. Kids love brownies, and these are a perfect addition to school lunches.

⅓	cup plus 1 tablespoon almond or peanut butter (almond butter can be found in health food stores)
½	cup granulated fructose
1	teaspoon vanilla
½	teaspoon salt
⅔	cup flour
110	grams of pure whey protein powder
⅓	cup unsweetened cocoa powder
1	cup water
1	tablespoon powdered sugar

Combine all ingredients in a 1-quart glass bowl and mix well. Batter will be rather thin.

Microwave on High for 2 minutes. Batter will be cooked around the edge and runny in the center. Remove from microwave and stir well. Return to microwave for 1 minute on High and stir well to blend. Batter should be moist but no longer runny, but microwaves can vary. If after stirring batter it is still runny, return to microwave for 20 to 40 additional seconds of cooking time. Overcooked batter will be very dry.

Scoop mixture into a buttered 8-inch-square pan. Mixture will be rather hot to touch, but while it is still hot, spread it evenly with a spoon. Cover with plastic wrap directly on brownie dough and continue to firmly press mixture evenly into pan with your hands. A clean towel can be placed on top of the plastic wrap if the dough is too hot to handle. Let cool.

Sift 1 tablespoon of powdered sugar on top of cooled brownies before serving. Cut into 16 slices.

Per slice: 120 calories; Grams = C-12g, P-9g, F-4g

CHOCOLATE ESPRESSO
BUNDT CAKE

*If you like coffee with chocolate cake, you are going to love
coffee in your cake. Instant espresso adds the unique flavor
and cream cheese provides the moist, rich texture. Don't serve
this cake chilled, as it's much better at room temperature.*

1	cup flour
100	grams of pure whey protein powder
2	teaspoons baking powder
½	teaspoon salt
½	cup cocoa powder
⅓	cup butter
16	ounces Philadelphia Brand Fat Free Cream Cheese
¾	cup granulated fructose
1	large egg
3	large egg whites
1	teaspoon vanilla
2	teaspoons instant coffee or espresso
⅓	cup nonfat milk
1	(1-ounce) square semisweet baking chocolate

Preheat oven to 300°F. Thoroughly grease and flour a 3-quart bundt pan. If
you miss a spot, the cake will stick.

Sift together flour, pure whey protein powder, baking powder, salt, and cocoa powder. Set aside.

Cream butter in a large mixing bowl. Add cream cheese and fructose and mix well. Add egg and egg whites, mixing well after each. Add vanilla.

In a small bowl, combine instant espresso powder with milk.

Add half of the flour mixture to the batter with half of the espresso-milk mixture and blend well; then add the remaining flour mixture and espresso milk and blend well.

Pour the batter into the prepared bundt pan and bake for 1 hour and 15 minutes or until a knife inserted into the center comes out clean. *Do not overbake* or cake will become dry. Remove from pan to cool on a wire rack. Cool cake completely before icing.

Melt the semisweet baking chocolate and drizzle it over the cake. Makes 24 servings.

Per serving: 115 calories; Grams = C-12g, P-9g, F-4g

Part Four

TROUBLESHOOTING

Chapter Twenty

ON THE ROAD

Travel, either for work or pleasure, requires relying completely on others to prepare your meals. Many people make travel an excuse for poor eating habits and complain that they have no control over what they are served, when in fact you choose from the menu and you pay the bill. Order what you want and insist they make it the way you want it. If a restaurant doesn't allow substitutions, feel free to go somewhere else.

BREAKFAST ON THE ROAD

Let's begin with breakfast. You've always heard that breakfast is the most important meal of the day. Actually, every meal is equally important. However, breakfast is the first meal of the day after you have fasted through the night. But, more important, breakfast should be thought of as your first opportunity to balance your blood sugar levels for the next four to five hours and elevate your fat burning hormone, glucagon. You have just programmed your body to burn fat as your primary source of energy.

Many hotels offer a continental breakfast, which usually consists of carbohydrate-rich foods like sweet rolls, cereal, bananas, juice, and coffee. If your choices consist only of high-carbohydrate foods, don't feel obligated to eat it just because it's free! We recently stayed at a hotel that offered cereal, sweet rolls, and juice, but also served fresh sliced fruit, yogurt, and a bowl of hard-boiled eggs.

Here is an example of the typical breakfast from a complimentary continental breakfast buffet:

	Calories	Carbs	Protein	Fat
1 banana	105	26.7	1.2	.6
1 box cornflakes	116	27	2	0
4 oz. lowfat milk	66	6.5	4	2.5
1 cherry cheese Danish	365	38	4	21
6 oz. orange juice	88	22	0	0
Total Calories	730	120 grams	11 grams	24 grams
		×4	×4	×9
		480 calories	44 calories	216 calories
PERCENTAGE OF CALORIES		66%	4%	30%

If you eat the above meal, 66% of the total calories are from carbohydrates, only 4% are from protein, and 30% are from fat. This meal will cause your blood sugar to spike and have you burning glucose rather than stored fat for energy, while excess calories will be converted into and stored as fat.

The following is an example of how to put together a Fat Flush Formula Meal from a breakfast buffet. This size is suitable for the C Plan:

	Calories	Carbs	Protein	Fat
2 whole hard-boiled eggs	145	1.2	12.6	10
3 hard-boiled eggs, whites only	51	.9	10.5	0
¾ cup fresh mixed fruit	128	32	0	0
½ cup yogurt, plain, lowfat	65	7.5	5.5	1.5
coffee or tea	0	0	0	0
Total Calories	389	41.6	29	11.5
		×4	×4	×9
		167	116	104
PERCENTAGE OF CALORIES		43%	30%	27%

The following is an example of how to choose a Regular Formula Meal from a breakfast buffet. This size is suitable for a C Plan:

	Calories	Carbs	Protein	Fat
2 whole hard-boiled eggs	145	1.2	12.6	10
3 hard-boiled eggs, whites only	51	.1	10.5	0
½ cup fresh mixed fruit	64	16	0	0
½ toasted English muffin	60	12	1	.2
½ teaspoon butter	9	0	0	1
coffee or tea	0	0	0	0
Total Calories	329	31.3	24.1	11.2
		×4	×4	×9
		152	96.4	100.8
PERCENTAGE OF CALORIES		39%	30%	31%

When eating breakfast in a sit-down restaurant, there are many variables. You may not be able to control portions or the amount of fat they cook with. Don't worry about your meals being perfect. Remember, close is good enough. Ask for dry toast or butter on the side, and if your omelette arrives covered in cheese or your toast is dripping with butter, return it for another order without cheese or butter.

The following are several examples of simple-to-order Fat Flush Formula and Regular Formula breakfasts. The sample meal portions listed are suitable for use with the A and B Personalized Meal Plans.

BREAKFAST
FAT FLUSH MEAL EXAMPLES

1. One whole egg and two egg whites with sliced tomato and fruit
2. Three eggs over easy (leave two yolks and eat all of the whites) with a bowl of fresh fruit
3. Denver omelette made with one egg and two whites with a bowl of fruit
4. Hot oatmeal with a side order of cottage cheese and strawberries

BREAKFAST
REGULAR MEAL EXAMPLES

1. Denver omelette made with one egg and two egg whites with 1 slice of whole wheat toast and jam
2. Scrambled eggs made with one egg and two egg whites with one slice of extra-lean ham and one pancake with one tablespoon syrup

3. Side order of extra-lean ham with one large or two medium pancakes and one tablespoon syrup

LUNCH ON THE ROAD

Approximately four to five hours after breakfast you'll need to refuel your body and stabilize your blood sugar for the next four hours by eating lunch. Listed here you will find options for lunches in a sit-down restaurant; please see page 203 for fast-food options.

When eating at a sit-down restaurant, begin by asking the server to remove (or not even bring) a basket of bread or chips. This way, these high-carbohydrate items won't be on the table tempting you.

The following are several examples of simple-to-order Fat Flush and Regular Formula lunch ideas. The sample meal portions are suitable for use with the C Personalized Meal Plan.

LUNCH

FAT FLUSH MEAL EXAMPLES

1. Grilled chicken Caesar salad without croutons with a large bowl of sliced fruit

2. Four ounces of tuna or chicken salad on a bed of lettuce with fresh sliced fruit

3. Grilled chicken or salmon with a

Fat Flush Meal Example

- *Salmon steak*
- *Steamed asparagus*
- *Artichoke*
- *Side salad with dressing*
- *Beverage (see* Appropriate Beverages)

large serving of steamed vegetables and a side salad with your favorite salad dressing on the side

Regular Meal Example:

- *Grilled fish or chicken (4- or 5-ounce serving)*
- *Rice*
- *Steamed vegetables*
- *Caesar salad with a few croutons*
- *Beverage*

LUNCH

REGULAR MEAL EXAMPLES

1. Grilled chicken Caesar salad with croutons and a four-ounce glass of wine
2. Grilled chicken Caesar salad without croutons with one slice of crusty French or sourdough bread (no butter)
3. Four ounces of sliced turkey on wheat, rye, or sourdough bread with lettuce, tomatoes, and mayonnaise with a dill pickle (no chips or fries)

SNACKS ON THE ROAD

You should eat again four hours after lunch to maintain stable blood sugar levels. This is typically the time most people start looking for something to snack on. Generally, only a small meal is needed at this time to control blood sugar for the next few hours until dinner.

If you skip the midafternoon snack and eat dinner at six or seven P.M., you can risk blood sugar dips and set yourself up for an out-of-control appetite at dinner. Don't expect lunch to control blood sugar levels for more than four or five hours. If you eat dinner at five P.M., you'll probably be fine.

But if you'll be up until ten P.M. or later, save your snack for four or five hours after dinner to be sure you have stable blood sugar before bed. Many clients who eat dinner early enjoy a 40-30-30 dessert as a late-night snack.

We generally rely on a 40-30-30 Nutrition Bar for our midafternoon snack. They are especially convenient when you are traveling and your choices are limited.

DINNER ON THE ROAD

When traveling, dinner in a nice restaurant means many choices. To begin with, ask your server to remove the basket of chips or bread (or not to bring them to the table at all). Request water and spend a little time reviewing the menu.

If you are using the Fat Flush Formula meals, follow these simple steps:

1. Choose one serving of a lowfat, high quality protein (chicken, beef, pork, or seafood)
2. Choose two large servings of low glycemic vegetables (broccoli, asparagus, green beans, mixed vegetable blend, or artichoke)
3. Choose a side salad with your favorite full-fat dressing on the side

If you are following the Regular Formula meals, follow these simple steps:

1. Choose one serving of a lowfat, high quality protein (chicken, beef, pork, or seafood)
2. Choose only one serving of a starchy food (potatoes, rice, pasta, or bread)
3. Choose one serving of vegetables
4. Choose a side salad with your favorite full-fat dressing on the side

If you plan to have an alcoholic beverage with your meal, count it as carbohydrates that should be part of the meal and reduce or eliminate the amount of starchy carbohydrates you order. Remember, it's the protein and fat in a meal that slows the digestion and absorption of the carbohydrates.

Alcoholic beverages can greatly vary in the amounts of carbohydrates and alcohol they contain. A light beer, a bloody Mary, or a glass of wine contains far less carbohydrates than a margarita, a mai tai, or a martini. A small margarita contains far less carbohydrates than a huge fishbowl-size margarita. The point is, if you drink alcoholic beverages, choose wisely and limit yourself to one. Then switch to water, sparkling water, or any other sugar-free beverage.

Should you decide to have an alcoholic beverage before your meal, have it with an appetizer that is high in protein with a small amount of fat and low in carbohydrates. Below are several examples for those eating Regular Meals.

REGULAR APPETIZER EXAMPLES

1. Four-ounce glass of wine with chicken strips
2. Martini with crab or shrimp cocktail
3. Margarita with a chicken-stuffed jalapeño pepper
4. Glass of beer with chicken skewers

5. Vodka tonic (or any mixed drink) with smoked salmon

6. Sake with beef-stuffed lettuce wraps

40-30-30 FAST-FOOD GUIDE

The majority of food found in fast-food restaurants contains too much fat and carbohydrates. However, we have found a variety of meals that contain an approximate 40-30-30 Formula. Below is a list you can use when you choose to eat fast food.

	Calories	Carb. Grams	Protein Grams	Fat Grams
Arby's (Light Menu)				
• Roast Beef Deluxe	296	33	18	10
• Roast Chicken Deluxe	276	33	20	6
• Roast Turkey Deluxe	260	33	20	7
Boston Market (Try these combinations)				
• Skinless Rotisserie Turkey Breast with Coleslaw, Steamed Vegetables, and Fruit Salad	470	53	41	21
• Rotisserie ¼ Chicken w/o skin with Broccoli Cauliflower AuGratin, Fruit Salad, Zucchini Marinara, and Green Beans	580	43	45	25.5
• Rotisserie ¼ Chicken w/o skin with Coyote Bean Salad, Tossed Salad w/ Fat Free Ranch Dressing, and Steamed Vegetables	470	61	44	16
• Rotisserie ¼ Chicken w/o skin with Butternut Squash, Green Beans, and Fruit Salad	480	47	37	15

	Calories	Carb. Grams	Protein Grams	Fat Grams
• Skinless Rotisserie Turkey Breast with Homestyle Mashed Potatoes and Gravy, Green Beans, and Fruit Salad	530	47	42	17.5
• Skinless Rotisserie Turkey Breast with Whole-Kernel Corn, Steamed Vegetables, and Broccoli Rice Casserole	625	64	48	17.5
• Skinless Rotisserie Turkey Breast with Savory Stuffing and Green Beans	560	50	43	19
• Rotisserie ¼ Chicken w/o skin with BBQ Baked Beans and Caesar Side Salad	640	57	48	26
• Rotisserie ¼ Chicken w/o skin with Macaroni and Cheese with Tossed Salad with Fat Free Ranch Dressing	610	63	51	17.5

Burger King
• BK Broiler Chicken Sandwich (order on hamburger bun)	315	30	26	10

Carl's Jr.
• BBQ Chicken Sandwich	280	37	25	3

Einstein/Noah Bagel
• ½ bagel with 4 oz. smoked salmon and 2 tablespoons cream cheese	450	42.5	30	18
• ½ bagel with turkey pastrami and 2 tablespoons cream cheese	340	40.5	27	8
• Tuna salad on baguette	305	36	26	10
• Harvest Chicken Salad on challah loaf	345	34	24	12.5
• Roast beef with 2 tablespoons mayonnaise on challah roll	420	40	28	15.5

	Calories	Carb. Grams	Protein Grams	Fat Grams
Jack in the Box				
• Chicken Fajitas Pita	320	34	24	10
• Grilled Chicken Fillet w/o mayonnaise	360	37	27	12
KFC				
• Tender Roast Chicken Sandwich	350	23	32	15
• Honey BBQ Flavored Chicken Sandwich	310	37	28	6
McDonald's				
• McGrilled Chicken Classic®	260	33	24	4
• Grilled Chicken Salad Deluxe with one packet Red French Reduced Calorie Dressing	280	30	21	9.5
Pizza Hut				
• Edge Pizza: Chicken/Veggie with double chicken (1 slice of a medium pie)	150	16	11	4
Subway				
• Super Subs: Subway Club with ½ tablespoon mayonnaise or olive oil blend	435	48	33	13
Taco Bell				
• Grilled Steak Soft Taco	200	19	14	7
• Grilled Chicken Soft Taco	200	20	14	7
Wendy's				
• Chili (small)	210	21	15	7
• Chili (large)	310	32	23	10
• Grilled Chicken Sandwich	300	36	24	8
• Spicy Chicken Sandwich w/o mayo	390	42	28	12

	Calories	Carb. Grams	Protein Grams	Fat Grams
• Chicken Caesar Fresh Stuffed Pitas®				
w/o dressing	410	47	30	12

Freshly Prepared Salads

	Calories	Carb. Grams	Protein Grams	Fat Grams
• Grilled Chicken Salad with	190	10	22	8
Italian (Reduced Fat, Reduced Calorie)	40	2	—	3
Soft Bread Stick	130	23	4	3
TOTAL	360	35	26	14
• Grilled Chicken Caesar Salad with	260	17	26	9
Soft Bread Stick	130	23	4	3
TOTAL	390	40	30	12

Wendy's Garden Spot Salad Bar (available in select restaurants only)

Try this combination:

	Calories	Carb. Grams	Protein Grams	Fat Grams
2 cups lettuce (iceberg/romaine)	24	4	2	0
Add one cup of mixed vegetables:				
(broccoli, cauliflower, mushrooms, tomato				
wedges, peppers, onions)	16	4	0	0
½ cup cottage cheese	120	4	16	6
⅓ cup diced eggs (mostly whites)	65	0	6	4
2 tablespoons bacon bits	45	0	6	2.5
2 tablespoons fat free dressing	30	8	0	0
½ cup sliced peaches w/ juice	60	16	0	0
TOTAL	360	40	30	12.5

Whataburger

	Calories	Carb. Grams	Protein Grams	Fat Grams
• Grilled Chicken Sandwich	420	48	34	14

The above nutrition information was derived from company brochures or Web sites. Variations may occur depending on the local supplier, the region of the country, and the season of the year. Some items may not be available at all locations. New product introductions or produce changes may cause deviations from the information listed in the tables.

EATING OUT, EVEN AT 7-ELEVEN

Listed below are a few examples of how you can follow the Formula even at 7-Eleven or convenience stores.

1. Lowfat cottage cheese and an apple, bottled water, and coffee or tea

2. Hard-boiled eggs and an orange with bottled water and coffee or tea

3. Balance 40-30-30 Nutrition Bars (1–2 whole bars) with bottled water and coffee or tea (we have worked with a lot of salespeople who have learned to rely on this example for a small high performance meal or snack that is a real time saver)

4. Chicken or chef salad with dressing and an apple with bottled water and a diet iced tea

5. Grilled chicken sandwich and raw veggies with dip with bottled water and a diet soda

6. Cottage cheese with raw mixed vegetables and dip with bottled water or sugar-free iced tea

7. Turkey pita pocket sandwich and an apple with bottled water and a diet soda

Chapter Twenty-one

HOW TO USE PREPACKAGED FOODS

Frozen meals and prepared foods have become popular due to our busy lifestyles. These meals are highly processed and high in sodium, so it is best to avoid them if you have been instructed to follow a low-sodium diet. The majority of prepared foods are predominantly high carbohydrate and high fat meals with a token amount of protein.

It is interesting to read the nutrition labels on prepared food. You'll find a variety of frozen and prepared foods ranging from lowfat to extra-large portions. Manufacturers that attempt to reduce fat to less than 10 grams per meal often end up reducing protein as well. These meals are generally far too high in carbohydrates:

Lowfat Meal Examples	Calories	Carbohydrates	Protein	Fat
Sweet and Sour Chicken Dinner	360	53	20	7
Mesquite Barbecue Chicken Dinner	310	48	18	5

The previous two examples contain approximately 15% of their total calories from fat. However, 60% of the total calories are from carbohydrates.

Manufacturers who make extra-large-portion meals typically make them very high in calories and load them with fat.

Extra-Large Meal Examples	Calories	Carbohydrates	Protein	Fat
Chicken Fried Steak Dinner	820	63	29	50
Salisbury Steak Dinner	780	47	27	54

The above two examples contain more than 55% of calories from fat and only about 14% from protein.

A simple way to determine if the nutrition profile of a prepared meal is close to the 40-30-30 Formula ratio is to begin by looking at the grams of protein. For example, use 21 grams of protein. The total carbohydrates should be one-third more. Divide 21 by 3 and add that total back to 21 grams (i.e.: $21 \div 3 = 7 + 21 = 28$ grams). Or you can multiply 21 grams $\times$ 1.33 = 27.93 grams. Either way, the carbohydrates would be 28 grams.

Where it gets tricky is determining the fat grams. Fat should be 30 percent of the total calories, so there are two ways to figure it out. The simplest way is to divide the grams of protein in half ($21 \div 2 = 10.5$). The fat should be just a little less than half of the protein. The more accurate way is to multiply the grams of protein times 4 to determine the total protein calories, then divide that number by 9 (i.e.: $21 \times 4 = 84 \div 9 = 9.33$).

IDEAL MEAL CONTAINING THE 40-30-30 FORMULA

Calories	Carbohydrate grams	Protein grams	Fat grams
280	28	21	9
	$\times 4$	$\times 4$	$\times 9$
	112	84	81 = 277 calories

Below are examples of prepared foods that are close enough to be used with the Formula's Regular Meals. Manufacturers are constantly changing and revising recipes, so please review the nutrition profile on the package when choosing your meals. The following breakdowns are per serving. You may need to have more than one serving to meet your requirements.

	Calories	Carb. Grams	Protein Grams	Fat Grams
Frozen and Prepared Meals				
Banquet Family				
• Beef with Noodles (1 cup)	150	16	11	5
Bridgford Micro-Ready				
• Chicken Breast Sandwich	320	34	23	10
Chef's Choice				
• Chicken Stir Fry	190	22	20	2
Fishery Products International				
• Caesar Salmon Pasta with Vegetables	170	23	14	3

	Calories	Carb. Grams	Protein Grams	Fat Grams
Freezer Queen Home Style				
• Beef with Potato and Carrots	160	19	15	3
• Beef with Gravy and Potatoes	140	17	14	2
Healthy Choice				
• Beef and Peppers	270	32	22	6
• Chicken Dijon	270	33	23	5
• Southwestern Chicken	260	30	21	6
• Chicken Picante	260	30	21	6
• Roasted Chicken Breast	230	23	20	6
Healthy Choice (Country Inn)				
• Roast Turkey	250	28	20	6
Healthy Choice Bowl Creations				
• Country Baked Chicken	230	22	18	8
Lean Cuisine (Cafe Classics)				
• Beef Peppercorn	220	23	15	7
• Beef Portobello	220	24	14	7
• Grilled Chicken	250	29	22	5
Lean Cuisine (American Favorites)				
• Salisbury Steak	280	29	24	8
• Chicken in Wine Sauce	210	23	15	6
• Glazed Chicken	240	25	22	6
Marie Callender's				
• Beef Tips in Mushroom Sauce	430	39	25	19
• Cheesy Rice and Chicken Breast	370	34	23	17
• Chicken Marsala	450	42	33	17
• Grilled Southwestern Style Chicken	410	43	34	11
• Roast Beef Dinner	390	30	24	19

	Calories	Carb. Grams	Protein Grams	Fat Grams
Smart Ones (Weight Watchers)				
• Grilled Salisbury Steak and Gravy	290	29	22	8
Stouffer's Skillet Sensations				
• Home Style Beef, ½ of 25-oz. packet	360	34	30	11
Tombstone Light Pizza				
• Supreme, ⅕ pie	270	30	25	9
• Vegetable, ⅕ pie	240	31	25	7
Tyson				
• Roasted Chicken with Garlic Sauce, Pasta, and Vegetables	210	20	17	7
Soup, Chili, and Stew				
Banquet Family				
• Beef Stew (1 cup)	160	17	14	4
Campbell's				
• Beef Vegetable	150	14	10	4
• Vegetable Won Ton	45	5	4	1
Dennison's				
• 99% Fat Free Beef Chili with Beans	220	27	22	2
Dinty Moore American Classics				
• Chow Mein, 1 bowl	270	28	22	8
• Turkey Chili, 1 bowl	290	32	22	8
Dinty Moore Microwave Cup				
• Chow Mein and Dumplings	200	21	15	6
Hunt's				
• Stew	155	20	14	4

	Calories	Carb. Grams	Protein Grams	Fat Grams
LaChoy, Bi-Pack				
• Chow Mein	100	10	8	4
Progresso				
• Beef Barley	130	13	10	4
• Beef Noodle	160	15	13	3.5
• Beef Vegetable and Rotini	130	14	13	2.5
• Hearty Chicken and Rotini	90	12	8	1.5
• Roasted Chicken Garden Herb	70	9	6	1.5
Wolf's				
• Lean Chili, 1 cup	200	21	15	8

FROZEN AND PREPARED FOOD TIPS

• If a meal contains more grams of fat than protein, don't buy it.

• If a meal contains more than twice as many carbohydrates as protein, you can adjust the ratio to equal the 40-30-30 Formula by adding sliced lean chicken, turkey, tuna, or any other lowfat protein.

• If a meal is too low in fat, add a small side salad with olive oil and vinegar salad dressing, or add nuts, avocados, or olives to increase the fat.

• Add steamed broccoli or another low glycemic vegetable or an apple or another low glycemic fruit when carbohydrates are too low.

• Avoid processed foods that are high in sodium if you have been advised to follow a low-sodium diet.

• If a meal contains the correct 40-30-30 Formula ratio but too few calories for your requirements, you may have to eat two servings. You can also add a serving of a 40-30-30 dessert.

Chapter Twenty-two

THE PARTY FORMULA

Holidays, parties, and special events mean entertaining with friends and food. But it shouldn't be a license to eat whatever you want. Parties are actually a great opportunity for you to practice your 40-30-30 skills.

If you are attending a cocktail party, survey the appetizers and choose from the high protein choices like meatballs, sushi, caviar, smoked salmon, shrimp, deviled eggs, or beef or chicken skewers, and have them with an alcoholic beverage, which will be your carbohydrates.

It is a good idea to eat a few protein appetizers before you begin drinking. The protein and fat found in the appetizers will help slow the absorption of alcohol and carbohydrates, helping to control the blood sugar surge alcoholic beverages can cause.

When you are hosting a cocktail party or special event, be sure to include several choices of lowfat protein for your guests to choose from. A variety of my favorite party foods includes a whole baked turkey, smoked salmon, pork tenderloin served with a variety of gourmet mustards, teriyaki chicken skewers, and cold cooked shrimp. Round out your table by including low glycemic fruits and vegetables such as a platter of whole strawberries and an assortment of sliced celery, baby carrots, cucumbers, and cherry tomatoes with a low-calorie vegetable dip plus a variety of gourmet olives.

One of my favorite clients entertained often and blamed her weight gain on too many parties. But after she'd been following the Formula and losing weight, the parties continued but the menus changed. Rather than preparing high-carbohydrate, high-fat appetizers, she now prepares an incredible assortment of light hors d'oeuvres that Martha Stewart would be proud of. Even her monthly ladies' day tea was transformed from fancy cookies and buttery sweet breads to elegant finger sandwiches and decadent 40-30-30 cheesecakes and biscotti.

Keep your social gathering healthy by providing your guests with balanced food choices and whatever they choose to drink.

Chapter Twenty-three

POWERFUL POINTERS

THE TOP TEN FORMULA TIPS
TO HELP BURN FAT FASTER

1. *Include protein every time you eat.* By including high quality protein in each meal, you can help stimulate the hormone glucagon. Glucagon can help keep blood sugar balanced and help you burn fat faster. Some of the best high quality, lowfat protein sources include 2% lowfat cottage cheese, eggs and egg whites, fish, chicken, turkey, beef and pork tenderloin, tofu, tempeh, and pure whey protein powder.

2. *Use primarily fruits and vegetables for your carbohydrate sources.* Low and medium glycemic fruits and vegetables will keep your blood sugar steady and control insulin. Some of the best low glycemic carbohydrate fruit sources include apples, cherries, oranges, peaches, grapes, pears, plums, and grapefruit. Vegetable sources include artichokes, asparagus, broccoli, cauliflower, celery, green beans, and salad greens. Fruits and vegetables are excellent sources of fiber, vitamins, and minerals.

3. *Don't be afraid of good fats.* Always include a serving of "good" fat at each meal. Good sources of fat can help balance blood sugar, control appetite, and provide essential fatty acids that are needed to help keep your hormones balanced. Some of the best sources of good fats include raw nuts and seeds such as almonds, walnuts, pecans, macadamia nuts, and sunflower seeds, as well as olives, olive oil, salmon and fish oil, and avocados. Use monounsaturated fats as your main source of fat and use saturated fats sparingly.

4. *Learn portion control.* Learn how to eat the right amount of food for your body size and activity level. The larger or more active you are, the more food you need. The smaller or less active you are, the less food you need. Even if your meals are balanced, a large meal containing excess calories can also increase insulin and contribute to weight gain just as much as excess carbohydrates can.

5. *Eat high fiber, low glycemic whole grains.* When using starchy carbohydrates use primarily high fiber, low glycemic sources, which are usually the most nutritious and also help control blood sugar. Their fiber content helps slow the digestion of the carbohydrates. Some of the best whole grain carbohydrate sources include barley, whole grain bread and pasta, rye, and brown and wild rice.

6. *Work your plan.* Use the appropriate personalized meal plan and all of the useful planning charts and guidelines that are included in this book.

Research has shown that when dieters are provided with and use detailed meal plans and a shopping list, they lose 50% more weight.

7. *Exercise.* Exercise at least 3 to 5 times per week. For the best results combine aerobic exercises, strength exercises, and stretching. Incorporate the 40-30-30 Exercise Formula.

8. *Hydrate.* Drink at least eight 8-ounce glasses of water each day. Burning fat is a dehydrating process. You can include fluids found in tea and coffee, but use pure water as your primary source of fluid. The more water you drink the better results you will get.

9. *Use meal supplements.* Instead of skipping meals, make following the 40-30-30 Formula even easier to stick to by using one of the 40-30-30 Nutrition Bars or drink mix powders that are now available. Also, pure whey protein powder can be used when making your own 40-30-30 smoothie. Don't miss meals. Eating every 4 to 5 hours ensures that your blood sugar will remain stable throughout the day.

10. *Read The Formula.* Since 1991 we have helped thousands of people use the 40-30-30 nutrition program. We have included everything you need to succeed in this book. So keep reading it again and again, because there is probably a solution in here for any problem that you might have. The Formula works; it has worked for us, for hundreds of thousands of our clients, and we know it can work for you.

MORE FORMULA TIPS

• *Deli meat hints.* When ordering sliced deli meats, order a pound of sliced deli meat but ask that they separate every 4 ounces with tissue so that it is premeasured for you. Then, when you need 4 ounces of meat it's already measured.

• *Buy a scale.* Purchase an inexpensive kitchen food scale. Use it often in the beginning to help you learn what three, four, or five ounces of raw or cooked protein looks like. After twenty-one days of practice, you will know amounts just by looking at them and you can put the scale away.

• *Buy measuring cups.* Stock your kitchen with a complete set of metal or plastic measuring cups to include ¼-, ⅓-, ½-, and 1-cup sizes.

• *Buy measuring spoons.* Stock your kitchen with a complete set of metal or plastic measuring spoons to include ⅛-, ¼-, ½-, and 1-teaspoon, plus ½- and 1-tablespoon sizes.

• *Use the palm of your hand.* Measure nuts using a measuring spoon, then place them in the palm of your hand before placing them in a recipe. Eventually you won't need to use the measuring spoon as you will automatically know proper amounts by using the palm of your hand.

• *Use fructose.* Fructose is a very low glycemic sweetener used in many of the recipes and desserts. Although sweeter than sugar, it is granulated, looks just like sugar, and can be found in most health food stores in the bulk section or in bags.

• *Use pure whey protein powder.* An excellent source of quality protein, pure whey protein powder is used in many recipes. It is derived from dairy, but is lactose and fat free and should contain no sweeteners or flavors. It mixes instantly, has no chalky aftertaste, and it can be found in most health food stores. Look for pure whey protein powder with the following nutritional profile:

PURE WHEY PROTEIN POWDER

Serving size:	1 scoop (22.2 grams)
Calories:	80
Carbohydrates:	0 grams
Protein:	20 grams
Fat:	0 grams

½ scoop = 5 grams, ⅓ scoop = 7 grams, ½ scoop = 10 grams,
⅔ scoop = 13 grams, ¾ scoop = 15 grams, 1 scoop = 20 grams

If you have trouble finding a pure whey protein, call Craig Nutraceuticals, Inc., at 1-800-293-1683. Ask for Pure WPI, by Bioplex Nutrition, the whey protein powder that the Daousts use in their recipes.

• *Close is good enough.* Meals don't have to contain the exact 40-30-30 ratio. 42-30-28, 39-31-30, 41-28-31, etc., are close enough. Food values differ from manufacturer to manufacturer, so meals will always differ. Just remember that close is good enough.

• *Avoid meals you don't like.* If there is a meal you don't like, don't eat it. There are plenty of delicious meals to choose from. Make only the meals that sound good to you. If a meal contains a fruit or vegetable you don't like, substitute a fruit or vegetable you do like.

• *Eat favorite meals often.* If you only like one breakfast out of all of those listed in this book, learn how to make it for your requirements and eat it every day. Most people have been eating the same bowl of cereal with juice and toast their entire life. Now you can switch to a 40-30-30 balanced breakfast instead.

• *Use 40-30-30 bars.* A typical 40-30-30 Nutrition Bar has been fortified with vitamins and minerals and should contain a profile similar to the following sample:

40-30-30 NUTRITION BAR

Calories:	190
Carbohydrates:	20 grams
Protein:	14 grams
Fat:	6 grams

• *Use 40-30-30 Shakes.* A typical 40-30-30 powder shake mix has been fortified with vitamins and minerals and should contain a profile similar to the following sample:

40-30-30 POWDER SHAKE MIX

Serving size:	2 scoops (43.2 grams)
Calories:	190
Carbohydrates:	20 grams
Protein:	14 grams
Fat:	6 grams

- *Use Emer'gen-C.* Used in several protein smoothie recipes, Emer'gen-C is a powdered vitamin C fizzy drink mix containing 32 mineral complexes. It is made by Alacer and can be found in most health food stores.

- *Use a Braun blender.* The Braun hand blender is our blender of choice when preparing smoothie recipes. If you don't have a blender, consider getting this one.

- *Substitutions.* If a meal contains a small amount of an item you don't like, such as onion in tuna salad, just leave it out. Omitting the few tablespoons of onion won't make a difference in carbohydrate content of the overall meal. If a meal contains 1 cup of asparagus and you don't like it, replace the asparagus with the same amount of another vegetable that is low glycemic, such as green beans or broccoli. The quantity of an item is what determines if it can be left out or if a substitution should be made.

- *Cooked meats.* When a recipe calls for cooked chicken, you will need about 20 to 25% more when buying raw chicken to be cooked. Five ounces of raw chicken will weigh about 4 ounces after it is cooked.

- *Salad Dressing.* If a recipe calls for oil and vinegar salad dressing, use any type of bottled dressing or just make your own. We use Paul Newman's Italian or Balsamic Vinegar and Olive Oil.

- *Try Prepackaged Spinach and Lettuce.* If you don't like to spend your time cleaning spinach and lettuce, buy it prepackaged in bags. It costs a little more, but it saves time and it's so convenient.

- *Eggs.* When a recipe calls for eggs, we always use large brown or white eggs (sometimes free-range or organic when available). We don't use egg substitutes. Fresh eggs are an inexpensive source of quality protein and we don't mind throwing the yolks out. You may want to hard-boil 6 to 12 eggs at a time to have on hand for a quick, ready-to-eat source of protein.

- *Use a butcher.* If you are cooking for more than one person, order an appropriate amount of protein from the butcher for both of you. For example, ask for one 5-ounce chicken breast and one 7-ounce chicken breast. Refer to the meal planners for the sizes you will need.

- *Cook Family Style.* Many of our recipes are Family Style Meals, usually soups, chili, and casseroles, and are great for the entire family. They can also be used as leftovers for lunch the next day or frozen for future dinners. Portion them out in the appropriate serving sizes before freezing.

- *Salad greens.* "Mixed salad greens" generally refers to dinner salads. If you only like one type of lettuce, use it. You can also add a few cherry tomatoes, chopped celery, onion, or other typical salad items. Use items that contain insignificant amounts of carbohydrates.

DID YOU KNOW . . .

THE SKINNY ON YOGURT

Did you know that many yogurts contain more sugar than a typical candy bar? The next time you are grocery shopping, stop by the yogurt display and check out the labels on several different yogurt cartons. This could take some time because the variety of choices has gotten rather large and includes fruit on the top or bottom, and sugar everywhere.

Now, while you're standing there browsing the labels, notice how many moms with children come by and fill their carts with these sugar-loaded treats. It's yogurt, the healthiest snack the kids will eat, right?

Maybe not. Take a closer look at some of the most popular yogurt flavors and you might be surprised at how high they are in carbohydrates, most of which is coming from added sugar. All of the examples listed below are lowfat or fat free, in 6-ounce sizes, and are national brands.

HIGH CARBOHYDRATE YOGURTS—6 OUNCE SERVINGS

	Calories	Carb.	Protein	Fat	% C, P, F
• Mixed berries	247	48	8	2.5	78-13-9
• Cherry, fruit on the bottom	243	45	9	3	74-15-11
• Chocolate cheesecake	221	45	8	1	81-14-5
• Pineapple	251	49	8	2.5	85-14-1
• Strawberry	176	36	8	0	82-18-0
• Vanilla caramel sundae	216	47	7	0	87-13-0

Instead of a high carbohydrate yogurt, make the following 40-30-30 Formula Yogurt Blend. You can convert many yogurts from a high sugar fat storing snack to a balanced, fat burning Formula meal. This is one of our favorite snack recipes that kids will love.

40-30-30 FORMULA YOGURT BLEND

	Calories	Carb.	Protein	Fat	% C, P, F
Yogurt Blend	245	27	20	7	42-31-26

Yogurt Blend
One fat-free yogurt (any flavor
  Knudsen Calorie 70)
¼ cup 2% cottage cheese
  (extra protein)
⅓ apple, sliced (good carbs)
1⅓ tablespoons sliced almonds
  (good fat)

DIRECTIONS: Combine the cottage cheese with yogurt and top with sliced apple and almonds.

SOY DRINKS

Did you know that many soy drinks are loaded with added sugar? In fact, quite a few contain more sugar than most soft drinks. If you use soy drinks, the next time you are shopping, take a few moments and check the labels on some of your favorite brands.

HIGH CARBOHYDRATE SOY DRINKS—8 OUNCES

	Calories	Carb.	Protein	Fat	% C, P, F
• Natural flavor, fat free	112	22	6	0	79-21-0
• Basic flavor, lowfat	118	20	4	1.5	75-14-11
• Carob flavor	213	36	7	4.5	67-13-20
• Vanilla flavor	147	24	6	3	65-16-18

The following is the breakdown of Soy Dream plain soy drink. It is still low in protein but will give you a better idea as to what you should look for when choosing soy drinks:

	Calories	Carb.	Protein	Fat	% C, P, F
• Soy Dream Original Flavor	133	14	6	5	42-24-34

Many people use soy drinks as a replacement for milk on breakfast cereals. The problem is that most cereals are very high in carbohydrates and low in protein and good fat. Adding a high carbohydrate cereal to the already high carbohydrate soy drink makes matters worse, because the entire meal is extremely high in carbohydrates. The solution is to simply add a little protein and fat to balance the carbohydrates. Below is a chart that shows you how to convert a high carbohydrate soy drink and cereal into a 40-30-30 Formula meal.

40-30-30 CEREAL WITH SOY MILK BREAKFAST

	Calories	Carb.	Protein	Fat	% C, P, F
Cereal with Soy Milk	335	34	25	11	40-30-30

1 cup Kellogg's All-Bran cereal
½ cup Soy Dream Original
    Flavor soy drink
15 grams pure whey protein powder
2 tablespoons sliced almonds

DIRECTIONS: Blend protein powder into soy drink, pour over cereal, and top with sliced almonds.

WHAT-IFS . . .

Different lifestyles result in a variety of situations, so for years we have been answering questions from thousands of people. We call them our What-Ifs. The following are the most commonly asked What-Ifs:

What if I'm planning on getting pregnant? You should certainly eat a balanced diet. The Formula provides balanced nutrition that will stabilize your blood sugar levels and improve your overall health and immune system.

What if I'm pregnant? Review the Formula with your doctor. Most doctors recommend that pregnant women eat a well-balanced diet, increasing calories by 25 to 30% in the second and third trimesters to supplement your additional nutritional needs. If you would normally follow the B plan, move to the C plan while pregnant as well as while breast-feeding.

What if I'm still hungry after a meal? If you are still hungry after any meal, first be sure that you made the meal correctly. For example, if you made a breakfast smoothie and forgot the nuts, you will be hungry very shortly thereafter. The nuts supply the fat that slows the digestion of the meal, helps to stabilize blood sugar, and controls your appetite for longer periods of time. If you are still hungry after certain meals, use the next larger meal plan. You may require slightly more calories at that meal or time of the day.

What if I can't eat all of the food? If the volume of a meal is too much and you cannot eat it all, you may be using too large a meal plan for your requirements. Drop down to the next smaller meal plan. Fat Flush meals contain a greater volume of carbohydrates due to the difference in density of low glycemic carbohydrates versus high glycemic carbohydrates. If Fat Flush Meals are too large, you can eat the majority of your meal and set aside the rest for an hour or two later. Be sure to save it in a balanced 40-30-30 portion.

What if I prefer to eat my larger meal at noon? The Formula meals were developed with breakfast being smaller in calories than lunch and lunch smaller than dinner only because most people have become accustomed to eating that way. If you prefer to eat a larger lunch and smaller dinner, you have several choices. You can switch the dinners for lunch. If you want to make your lunch meals larger, you need to refer to the Macronutrient Chart on page 276. If you are following the C plan, lunches contain 40 grams of carbohydrates, 30 grams of protein, and 14 grams of fat. Dinners contain 53 grams of carbohydrates, 40 grams of protein, and 18 grams of fat. To increase a lunch size and decrease a dinner, use the D amount for lunch and the A amount for dinner.

What if I work the graveyard shift? When your work schedule differs from the "norm," simply determine when you eat your first meal of the day after waking and consider that breakfast. Be certain to eat every 4 to 5 hours to maintain stable blood sugar levels throughout the day.

What if I don't like certain foods? Don't eat meals that contain foods you don't like. There are many meals to choose from. Eat only the meals that appeal to you.

What if I'm allergic to certain foods? Avoid any meals that contain foods you cannot eat. You may also substitute a particular food you may be allergic to, such as strawberries, for an alternative source, like peaches. Just remember to substitute a low glycemic carbohydrate for another low glycemic carbohydrate, and so on.

What if my kids are really picky eaters? Through the years, we have found many meals kids like and marked them Kids' Favorites. Review all of the meals and find a few meals your kids like and make them often. A woman with five picky children called to tell us she was thrilled that all of her children loved the pizza and Sloppy Joe recipes. She commented that she once made the Sloppy Joe recipe five days in a row.

If your kids are used to sweet cereals in the morning, choose the fruit smoothies or 40-30-30 Nutrition Bars instead. These taste sweet but follow the 40-30-30 Formula to help stabilize blood sugar levels rather than spike them.

What if I'm single but want to use the Family Style meals? Family Style meals can easily be divided into exact portions and frozen. Three lady friends on the C Plan told us how they each would make a different Family Style meal recipe, divide them into appropriate serving portions, and split them between themselves for variety without all the cooking. You might also consider dividing them into smaller amounts for lunch portions.

What if I have high blood pressure? The Formula helps stabilize blood sugar, controls insulin, and helps prevent the constriction of blood vessels, thus reducing your risk of and helping to control high blood pressure.

What if I don't eat lunch until later in the afternoon and dinner rather early? If your lunch break isn't until 1:30 and you eat dinner between 5:30 and 6:00, you may not need the midafternoon snack. However, since lunch is late, if breakfast is eaten at 7:00 A.M., you should have a snack four hours later to prevent blood sugar dips in the morning. Just remember that meals can help to stabilize blood sugar levels for about 4 hours, snacks for about 2 hours.

What if the scale isn't changing but my clothes are looser? We hear this more often from women, who don't know if they should be glad or upset. Many diets promise weight loss while sacrificing lean muscle mass and slowing the metabolism. With this in mind, when a woman who is muscle wasted begins to use the Formula, muscle mass is regained while losing only body fat. Don't worry about the scale. You are losing unwanted body fat and gaining precious lean muscle mass, improving muscle tone and strength throughout your body. If a woman loses 2 pounds of fat but gains 2 pounds of muscle, the scale doesn't change. We often hear the comment that muscle weighs more than fat. However, one pound of muscle weighs the same as one pound of fat. A pound is a pound. The difference is in the *size* of a pound of muscle versus that of a pound of fat. One pound of muscle is quite a bit smaller than one pound of fat. Put away your scale and use a tape measure or body-fat calipers to monitor your results. Your body will be getting smaller, more toned, and fit, and you will love what you see in the mirror.

What if I plateau? If you have been following the Regular Formula Meals and hit a plateau, switch to the Fat Flush Formula Meals and increase your activity level. You haven't really hit a plateau. You are still losing body fat and increasing lean muscle mass. We worked with a man who was 5 feet 11 inches, weighed 190 pounds, and had 22% body fat when he began following the Formula and exercising. In four months, his weight was still 190 pounds, but his body fat had dropped to 10%. He was thrilled. At 22% body fat, a 190-pound man has 42 pounds of body fat and 148 pounds of lean body mass. At 10% body fat, a 190-pound man has only 19 pounds of body fat and 171 pounds of lean body mass. He actually lost 23 pounds of pure fat while gaining 23 pounds of lean muscle mass. The scale stayed the same—it was his entire wardrobe that changed.

What if it doesn't work for me? If the Formula doesn't work for you, you haven't been following it. A woman swore she was following the program but seeing no results. We asked her to describe her meals. We were curious when it appeared she was following the meals. It was only when we asked what she drank that we discovered she drank coffee with sugar all morning, several sodas a day, and sucked on hard candy. When we added up the extra sugar calories, she was far over in carbohydrates. Even though her meals were perfectly balanced, the in-between-meal high carbohydrate drinks and candy were spiking blood sugar and preventing her from losing body fat. Two days later we heard from her again. She dropped 7 pounds. How can that be? High carbohydrate diets spike blood sugar and elevate insulin levels to lower it. Insulin is a storage hormone and can cause water retention and bloating. When she eliminated the extra carbohydrates, her blood sugar stabilized, reducing insulin and allowing her body to dump the excess fluids she had been retaining. She commented that her rings fit looser and her shoes fit better. It didn't take long for her to realize the Formula works for everyone, but only if you use it correctly.

What if I exercise in the morning? Most people have stable blood sugar when they wake and should eat within an hour after waking to keep it that way. If you wake up and immediately begin to exercise without eating a balanced meal, you risk blood sugar dropping during exercise, experiencing an energy slump, and not getting the most from your workout. But training on a full stomach isn't the answer either. When we work out first thing in the morning, we get up, drink a glass of water, and eat one-third to one-half of a 40-30-30 Nutrition Bar. The water hydrates our bodies while the small

̶ ̶ ̶ ̶ ̶ ̶ ̶ digested and ensures our blood sugar level and en-

at breakfast within

for the next 4 to 5

fast around 8 A.M.

pply a small source

rkout. Eat a small

d to one-half of a

s your body, while

o digest and keeps

ve better access to

ut. Eat lunch after

te a portion of your

snack two to three

e your midafternoon

are balanced during

e for your brain. Eat

snack if dinner will

What if I'm an advanced athlete? The more active you are, the more food you need to fuel your highly trained muscles. There are several variables to choosing the appropriate meal plan for athletic requirements. A woman weighing 125 pounds who is active would normally use the B Meal Plan. A competitive female athlete swimmer, volleyball player, or soccer player, for example, should use the C Meal Plan on days activity levels are at their peak and during training and competition. A larger, highly trained female athlete who weighs 160 pounds may need to use the D Meal Plan during peak training and competition. Men who would normally require the C or D Meal Plan should follow the E plan when training or during competition.

What if I exercise and have a physical job? A man following the Formula using the D plan was losing weight but complaining that he was still getting hungry during the day. We discovered he was a UPS driver and lifting weights five days per week. His activity was equal to that of an advanced athlete and he required additional calories to fuel that activity. We moved him to the E Meal Plan and his hunger was controlled and his energy levels improved. If you don't eat enough food for your size and activity level, fat loss slows and energy levels suffer.

What if I don't exercise at all? We love to exercise. It's just part of our lifestyle. But we realize there are many people who don't like to exercise or claim to have no time for exercise. An Ob/Gyn in San Diego did a four-week study of twenty-two women using our Fat Flush program. They were instructed to exercise thirty minutes per day, but at the end of the four weeks, twenty of the twenty-two women admitted they didn't do the required exercise. They still saw impressive results in weight loss without muscle loss, increased energy levels, and improved cholesterol, blood pressure, and fasting glucose levels. When you follow the Formula, you burn fat as your primary source of energy. Exercise will increase the fat burning process and give you even better results.

What if I eat out all of the time? Many people eat out on a regular basis. This requires relying on others to prepare your meals. Choose meals from the menu that are similar to those found in this book. If your meal arrives with enough carbohydrates to feed a family of four, eat only enough for your requirements and leave the rest. Refer to our Fast Food and Dining Out recommendations for meal samples.

What if I don't cook? Many people don't cook but still follow the Formula. 40-30-30 Nutrition Bars and Shakes can eliminate the need for several meals or snacks each day. Refer to our Fast Food and Dining Out recommendations for meal samples. Many lowfat frozen dinner entrees come close to the 40-30-30 ratio. If a frozen dinner entree contains 30 grams of protein, 40 grams of carbohydrates, but only 5 grams of fat, it can easily be adjusted. While heating the frozen meal, prepare a side salad with enough salad dressing to equal 9 grams of fat.

What if desserts are my downfall? You are in luck. Studies show that if you deprive people of sweet treats and desserts, they quickly give up a restrictive diet. So why restrict sweets when you can enjoy them on the Formula? The 40-30-30 Nutrition Bars and Shakes taste sweet but contain low glycemic sweeteners and include protein and fat. The protein and fat are the important components that control carbohydrate metabolism.

The Formula provides delicious recipes for cheesecakes, puddings, cakes, cookies, and more that are 40-30-30 compatible and can be eaten as a snack during the day or for an occasional after-dinner dessert. Granulated fructose, a low glycemic sweetener, replaces sugar, pure whey protein powder is used to fortify protein needs, and fat is reduced to only 30 percent of every recipe. So whether you eat a 40-30-30 balanced meal for breakfast, a 40-30-30 Nutrition Bar, or even a slice of the Formula cheesecake, as long as it's the 40-30-30 Formula, you can help your body stimulate the production of glucagon, the key to getting rid of unwanted body fat while keeping blood sugar steady and energy high from meal to meal.

Part Five

MOTIVATIONAL TOOLS

Chapter Twenty-four

DOES THIS
SOUND LIKE YOU?

Y ou exercise like crazy, watch what you eat, but still can't seem to lose the weight you want. Or maybe you simply want to feel and perform better. Well, the Formula is not just for losing weight; it is a balanced eating plan for everyone. We truly believe the Formula with its 40-30-30 caloric ratio is the greatest breakthrough ever in nutrition. It worked for us and for thousands of our clients, and we know it can work for you.

Through the years we have helped hundreds of thousands of people use the Formula and have seen it work on all types of individuals, from housewives to truck drivers, competitive athletes to corporate executives.

Listed below are several stories of how the Formula has helped us and other individuals. They may give you some insight into how the Formula can help you.

A STORY ABOUT HUNGER

Gene's story began when he was a kid. He was overweight as a child and struggled to control his weight with athletics. Although sports helped to manage his weight problem, he was consumed by hunger. Like many athletes, a ravenous appetite began to control his life. While eating breakfast he was often planning his next meal.

But in 1990, he learned about the 40-30-30 ratio and for the first time ever was able to control his hunger from meal to meal. Constant hunger was a thing of the past. Not only did the Formula control his hunger, but he lost 15 pounds of pure body fat and has kept it off. He didn't have to give up his favorite foods; he simply learned how to eat a balanced diet that regulated the hormones to control hunger, burn fat, and build lean muscle mass.

A LOVE STORY

Joyce's personal story is about love—her love of carbohydrates. Having struggled with a weight problem most of her life, she bought into the misconception that fat was bad and carbohydrates were good. She jogged and did aerobics for one and a half to two hours every morning, then ate a large bowl of oatmeal with raisins and brown sugar. But by 11 A.M., her blood sugar levels would drop so severely, headaches, dizziness, and fatigue would consume her. It was so intense that only M&M candies seemed to relieve it. She always carried a bag in her purse. Her blood sugar levels would rise, relieving some of the hypoglycemic symptoms, which would only return again a few hours later, leaving her sleepy and fatigued.

In 1990, after she learned about the 40-30-30 ratio, her life changed forever. After her very first 40-30-30 balanced breakfast, her blood sugar levels stabilized. She couldn't believe how in control she felt, while her energy levels soared and her PMS cravings and cramps disappeared— along with 10 pounds of fat and the cellulite on the back of her legs.

Her transformation changed her love for carbohydrates to the love of a balanced diet and an intense desire to share this revelation with others.

A TWELVE-YEAR-OLD'S STORY

John is our twelve-year-old nephew and a good athlete. Like most kids, he likes junk food, and after school before sports practice he would practically inhale cookies, chips, and peanut butter and jelly sandwiches. He also thinks the world of his uncle Gene, who informed him that all those carbohydrates weren't doing anything to improve his athletic performance. His mom started giving him the option of a 40-30-30 Balance Bar before practice or games. It didn't take long for him to realize that his focus had improved, his energy was steadier and he was quickly becoming "the bomb."

Now he won't eat anything but a bar before his games to keep him focused and in the zone. His coaches have noticed a huge improvement and so have his teammates. Now they all want to eat his bars.

A SALES STORY

Kevin is a computer sales representative who works in New Jersey and New York. Being a competitive guy with huge quotas to meet, he found himself flying out of the house each morning, relying on coffee from

7-Eleven to get him through the day. By the evening, he was completely fatigued, starving, and would eat everything in sight. Although he ate only one huge meal a day, his weight was creeping up while his energy levels were declining.

He met with Gene, who explained the importance of balanced meals throughout the day. He began keeping 40-30-30 Balance Bars and bottled water in his car at all times. Rather than missing breakfast and lunch, he would grab a bar with coffee or water. In just a few days he noticed improved energy and focus. As his body fat dropped, his sales went up, and soon he was meeting and exceeding quotas and goals. Rather than eating all evening, he found time for a workout at the gym.

A PRIVATE STORY

Pete is a private trainer in the San Diego area. He was recognized by *Vogue* magazine as one of the top trainers in the world. Having trained thousands of individuals for years, he embraced the concept of the Formula. It provided him with the missing link his clients needed to achieve the results they expected.

A successful training program should include exercise as well as a balanced 40-30-30 diet.

A FAMILY AFFAIR

Betsy and Craig are a married couple who led a lethargic lifestyle as the largest people in a small town. After several diets failed her, Betsy heard of the 40-30-30 Formula and decided it made sense enough to try. The Formula changed their lives. They each lost more than 100 pounds and tapped into a powerful source of energy. Now they are two of the most fit, active, and energetic people in their small town.

A LIFESAVING STORY

Steve was suffering from ALS (Lou Gehrig's disease), completely immobile, and losing weight at an alarming rate. His wife contacted us for help. We went to their home to discover a 96-pound former triathlete, wasting away. We asked his 24-hour nursing staff what they were feeding him and were alarmed to see several cans of a popular medical meal replacement drink.

The muscle loss stopped that day with a completely balanced diet. Since everything had to be liquid to fit through a feeding tube, we pulled out the blender and began to design 40-30-30 meals out of jars of baby food. Within days his energy was improving, and after a year his weight was up to 135 pounds. The nurses exercised his muscles several times a day and would comment on their improved tone and size. The weight gain was mostly muscle. If the nurses didn't prepare the meals correctly, Steve would let them know he felt bad and they would adjust his next meal. A balanced diet eaten at every meal stimulates the production of glucagon and improves access to growth hormone, thus eliminating muscle wasting, building lean muscle mass, and keeping energy and concentration high.

Steve is still in a wheelchair waiting for researchers to discover new technology for nerve regeneration. But now while he continues his wait, his balanced diet has definitely improved the quality of his life.

A HAIR-SAVING STORY

Cheryl is a woman who phoned us one day to express her gratitude for the 40-30-30 Formula. She told us how she had been on diets all her life. In fact, she was the bookkeeper for a well-known nationwide diet center: not only had these diets not been successful, they were low in protein, which caused her body proteins to break down, resulting in hair loss. After attending a seminar we presented, she decided the 40-30-30 Formula made sense. After two months on the Fat Flush program, she wanted to tell us that for the first time in her life, she had lost weight without losing her hair.

A GREAT NEWS STORY

Belinda is a journalist in a small town who initially wanted to write a story on the 40-30-30 Formula diet. Her idea was to follow someone through the diet program. After she read our first book, it made so much sense to her, she chose herself. Within six months, she lost forty-six pounds and went from a size eighteen to a size ten, then continued on to a size eight. She had rave reviews for the Family Style meals her entire family could enjoy. Precise meal plans kept her on track in the beginning and taught her how to judge pretty much any meal. As a busy journalist, she raved about her new-found energy levels and is most proud of having been able to influence hundreds of people in her town through her personal experience.

Chapter Twenty-five

PLANNING GUIDES

I t has been said that if you fail to plan, you are planning to fail. With that in mind, we have designed two tracking journals that are easy-to-use and powerful tools to help you achieve your goals and track your results.

21-DAY FAT FLUSH
STAR TRACKER

This is a unique, self-motivating personal nutrition journal. Simply write down what you eat and drink and give yourself a star when appropriate. The object is to obtain ten stars each day as often as possible. You will be amazed at how well this journal works. It's like having your own personal nutrition coach. After you have used the journal and achieved results, keep it as a reference guide for the future. We have included a sample page of the 21-Day Fat Flush Star Tracker to help you get started.

FORMULA FOR LIFE
MONTHLY TRACKER

This guide will help you keep track of all of the great results you can achieve when following the Formula for the rest of your life. Through the years we have heard thousands of unbelievable success stories. Once a month, weigh and measure yourself and fill in the blanks with the results you are having. Upon regular visits to your doctor, jot down your blood pressure, cholesterol, HDL, LDL, and body-fat percentage. You will be able to track the results of your new lifestyle while improving the quality of your life.

_____
(Your name)

21 DAY FAT FLUSH STAR TRACKER

This convenient 21-Day Fat Flush Star Tracker is a nutrition journal to help keep you motivated and assist you in reaching your goals. For the next 21 days, give yourself a star for each Fat Flush Formula meal you eat and jot down a brief description of the meal. Give yourself another star every time you drink 8 ounces of water or more. The goal is to record ten stars per day. At the bottom of the page, you may want to jot down any thoughts or feelings regarding hunger, favorite meals, energy levels, moods, etc.

Day 1 of 21

Today's date: *1/1/01*

BREAKFAST: Record your meal and give yourself a star for a Fat Flush Formula meal and if you drank 8 or more ounces of water. *Eggs and Fruit*

Fat Flush meal star ⭐ 8 ounces of water star ⭐ Stars = *2*

LUNCH: Record your meal and give yourself a star for a Fat Flush Formula meal and if you drank 8 or more ounces of water. *Tuna Stuffed Tomato*

Fat Flush meal star ⭐ 8 ounces of water star ⭐ Stars = *2*

SNACK: Record your meal and give yourself a star for a Fat Flush Formula meal and if you drank 8 or more ounces of water. *Balance Bar*

Fat Flush meal star ⭐ 8 ounces of water star ⭐ Stars = *1*

DINNER: Record your meal and give yourself a star for a Fat Flush Formula meal and if you drank 8 or more ounces of water. *Beef Barley Soup*

Fat Flush meal star ⭐ 8 ounces of water star ⭐ Stars = *2*

EXERCISE: Describe your workout and give yourself a star for exercising and if you had 8 ounces or more of water. *Walked, Did Weights, and Stretched*

Exercised ⭐ 8 ounces of water star ⭐ Stars = *2*

NOTES: Record the total stars you achieved for the day, how you felt, and any notes: *Need to up the water. I'm feeling great!*

TODAY'S TOTAL STARS = *9*

Good job and congratulations, you're a STAR!

(Your name)

21 DAY FAT FLUSH STAR TRACKER

This convenient 21-Day Fat Flush Star Tracker is a nutrition journal to help keep you motivated and assist you in reaching your goals. For the next 21 days, give yourself a star for each Fat Flush Formula meal you eat and jot down a brief description of the meal. Give yourself another star every time you drink 8 ounces of water or more. The goal is to record ten stars per day. At the bottom of the page, you may want to jot down any thoughts or feelings regarding hunger, favorite meals, energy levels, moods, etc.

Day 1 of 21
Today's date: _____/_____/_____

BREAKFAST: Record your meal and give yourself a star for a Fat Flush Formula meal and if you drank 8 or more ounces of water.

Fat Flush meal star ☆ 8 ounces of water star ☆ Stars = ☆

LUNCH: Record your meal and give yourself a star for a Fat Flush Formula meal and if you drank 8 or more ounces of water.

Fat Flush meal star ☆ 8 ounces of water star ☆ Stars = ☆

SNACK: Record your meal and give yourself a star for a Fat Flush Formula meal and if you drank 8 or more ounces of water.

Fat Flush meal star ☆ 8 ounces of water star ☆ Stars = ☆

DINNER: Record your meal and give yourself a star for a Fat Flush Formula meal and if you drank 8 or more ounces of water.

Fat Flush meal star ☆ 8 ounces of water star ☆ Stars = ☆

EXERCISE: Describe your workout and give yourself a star for exercising and if you had 8 ounces or more of water.

Exercised ☆ 8 ounces of water star ☆ Stars = ☆

NOTES: Record the total stars you achieved for the day, how you felt, and any notes:

TODAY'S TOTAL STARS = ☆

Good job and congratulations, you're a STAR!

_____
(Your name)

21 DAY FAT FLUSH STAR TRACKER

This convenient 21-Day Fat Flush Star Tracker is a nutrition journal to help keep you motivated and assist you in reaching your goals. For the next 21 days, give yourself a star for each Fat Flush Formula meal you eat and jot down a brief description of the meal. Give yourself another star every time you drink 8 ounces of water or more. The goal is to record ten stars per day. At the bottom of the page, you may want to jot down any thoughts or feelings regarding hunger, favorite meals, energy levels, moods, etc.

Day 2 of 21
Today's date: ____/____/____

BREAKFAST: Record your meal and give yourself a star for a Fat Flush Formula meal and if you drank 8 or more ounces of water.

Fat Flush meal star ⭐ 8 ounces of water star ⭐ Stars = ⭐

LUNCH: Record your meal and give yourself a star for a Fat Flush Formula meal and if you drank 8 or more ounces of water.

Fat Flush meal star ⭐ 8 ounces of water star ⭐ Stars = ⭐

SNACK: Record your meal and give yourself a star for a Fat Flush Formula meal and if you drank 8 or more ounces of water.

Fat Flush meal star ⭐ 8 ounces of water star ⭐ Stars = ⭐

DINNER: Record your meal and give yourself a star for a Fat Flush Formula meal and if you drank 8 or more ounces of water.

Fat Flush meal star ⭐ 8 ounces of water star ⭐ Stars = ⭐

EXERCISE: Describe your workout and give yourself a star for exercising and if you had 8 ounces or more of water.

Exercised ⭐ 8 ounces of water star ⭐ Stars = ⭐

NOTES: Record the total stars you achieved for the day, how you felt, and any notes:

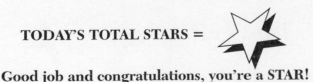

TODAY'S TOTAL STARS =

Good job and congratulations, you're a STAR!

21 DAY FAT FLUSH STAR TRACKER

This convenient 21-Day Fat Flush Star Tracker is a nutrition journal to help keep you motivated and assist you in reaching your goals. For the next 21 days, give yourself a star for each Fat Flush Formula meal you eat and jot down a brief description of the meal. Give yourself another star every time you drink 8 ounces of water or more. The goal is to record ten stars per day. At the bottom of the page, you may want to jot down any thoughts or feelings regarding hunger, favorite meals, energy levels, moods, etc.

Day 3 of 21
Today's date: _____/_____/_____

BREAKFAST: Record your meal and give yourself a star for a Fat Flush Formula meal and if you drank 8 or more ounces of water.

Fat Flush meal star ⭐   8 ounces of water star ⭐   Stars = ⭐

LUNCH: Record your meal and give yourself a star for a Fat Flush Formula meal and if you drank 8 or more ounces of water.

Fat Flush meal star ⭐   8 ounces of water star ⭐   Stars = ⭐

SNACK: Record your meal and give yourself a star for a Fat Flush Formula meal and if you drank 8 or more ounces of water.

Fat Flush meal star ⭐   8 ounces of water star ⭐   Stars = ⭐

DINNER: Record your meal and give yourself a star for a Fat Flush Formula meal and if you drank 8 or more ounces of water.

Fat Flush meal star ⭐   8 ounces of water star ⭐   Stars = ⭐

EXERCISE: Describe your workout and give yourself a star for exercising and if you had 8 ounces or more of water.

Exercised ⭐   8 ounces of water star ⭐   Stars = ⭐

NOTES: Record the total stars you achieved for the day, how you felt, and any notes:

TODAY'S TOTAL STARS = ⭐

Good job and congratulations, you're a STAR!

_____

(Your name)

21 DAY FAT FLUSH STAR TRACKER

This convenient 21-Day Fat Flush Star Tracker is a nutrition journal to help keep you motivated and assist you in reaching your goals. For the next 21 days, give yourself a star for each Fat Flush Formula meal you eat and jot down a brief description of the meal. Give yourself another star every time you drink 8 ounces of water or more. The goal is to record ten stars per day. At the bottom of the page, you may want to jot down any thoughts or feelings regarding hunger, favorite meals, energy levels, moods, etc.

Day 4 of 21

Today's date: ____/____/____

BREAKFAST: Record your meal and give yourself a star for a Fat Flush Formula meal and if you drank 8 or more ounces of water.

Fat Flush meal star ⭐ 8 ounces of water star ⭐ Stars = ⭐

LUNCH: Record your meal and give yourself a star for a Fat Flush Formula meal and if you drank 8 or more ounces of water.

Fat Flush meal star ⭐ 8 ounces of water star ⭐ Stars = ⭐

SNACK: Record your meal and give yourself a star for a Fat Flush Formula meal and if you drank 8 or more ounces of water.

Fat Flush meal star ⭐ 8 ounces of water star ⭐ Stars = ⭐

DINNER: Record your meal and give yourself a star for a Fat Flush Formula meal and if you drank 8 or more ounces of water.

Fat Flush meal star ⭐ 8 ounces of water star ⭐ Stars = ⭐

EXERCISE: Describe your workout and give yourself a star for exercising and if you had 8 ounces or more of water.

Exercised ⭐ 8 ounces of water star ⭐ Stars = ⭐

NOTES: Record the total stars you achieved for the day, how you felt, and any notes:

TODAY'S TOTAL STARS = ⭐

Good job and congratulations, you're a STAR!

_____

(Your name)

21 DAY FAT FLUSH STAR TRACKER

This convenient 21-Day Fat Flush Star Tracker is a nutrition journal to help keep you motivated and assist you in reaching your goals. For the next 21 days, give yourself a star for each Fat Flush Formula meal you eat and jot down a brief description of the meal. Give yourself another star every time you drink 8 ounces of water or more. The goal is to record ten stars per day. At the bottom of the page, you may want to jot down any thoughts or feelings regarding hunger, favorite meals, energy levels, moods, etc.

Day 5 of 21

Today's date: ____/____/____

BREAKFAST: Record your meal and give yourself a star for a Fat Flush Formula meal and if you drank 8 or more ounces of water.

Fat Flush meal star ⭐ 8 ounces of water star ⭐ Stars = ⭐

LUNCH: Record your meal and give yourself a star for a Fat Flush Formula meal and if you drank 8 or more ounces of water.

Fat Flush meal star ⭐ 8 ounces of water star ⭐ Stars = ⭐

SNACK: Record your meal and give yourself a star for a Fat Flush Formula meal and if you drank 8 or more ounces of water.

Fat Flush meal star ⭐ 8 ounces of water star ⭐ Stars = ⭐

DINNER: Record your meal and give yourself a star for a Fat Flush Formula meal and if you drank 8 or more ounces of water.

Fat Flush meal star ⭐ 8 ounces of water star ⭐ Stars = ⭐

EXERCISE: Describe your workout and give yourself a star for exercising and if you had 8 ounces or more of water.

Exercised ⭐ 8 ounces of water star ⭐ Stars = ⭐

NOTES: Record the total stars you achieved for the day, how you felt, and any notes:

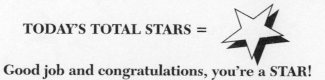

TODAY'S TOTAL STARS =

Good job and congratulations, you're a STAR!

_____
(Your name)

21 DAY FAT FLUSH STAR TRACKER

This convenient 21-Day Fat Flush Star Tracker is a nutrition journal to help keep you motivated and assist you in reaching your goals. For the next 21 days, give yourself a star for each Fat Flush Formula meal you eat and jot down a brief description of the meal. Give yourself another star every time you drink 8 ounces of water or more. The goal is to record ten stars per day. At the bottom of the page, you may want to jot down any thoughts or feelings regarding hunger, favorite meals, energy levels, moods, etc.

Day 6 of 21

Today's date: ____/____/____

BREAKFAST: Record your meal and give yourself a star for a Fat Flush Formula meal and if you drank 8 or more ounces of water.

Fat Flush meal star ⭐   8 ounces of water star ⭐   Stars = ⭐

LUNCH: Record your meal and give yourself a star for a Fat Flush Formula meal and if you drank 8 or more ounces of water.

Fat Flush meal star ⭐   8 ounces of water star ⭐   Stars = ⭐

SNACK: Record your meal and give yourself a star for a Fat Flush Formula meal and if you drank 8 or more ounces of water.

Fat Flush meal star ⭐   8 ounces of water star ⭐   Stars = ⭐

DINNER: Record your meal and give yourself a star for a Fat Flush Formula meal and if you drank 8 or more ounces of water.

Fat Flush meal star ⭐   8 ounces of water star ⭐   Stars = ⭐

EXERCISE: Describe your workout and give yourself a star for exercising and if you had 8 ounces or more of water.

Exercised ⭐   8 ounces of water star ⭐   Stars = ⭐

NOTES: Record the total stars you achieved for the day, how you felt, and any notes:

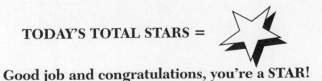

TODAY'S TOTAL STARS = ⭐

Good job and congratulations, you're a STAR!

_____

(Your name)

21 DAY FAT FLUSH STAR TRACKER

This convenient 21-Day Fat Flush Star Tracker is a nutrition journal to help keep you motivated and assist you in reaching your goals. For the next 21 days, give yourself a star for each Fat Flush Formula meal you eat and jot down a brief description of the meal. Give yourself another star every time you drink 8 ounces of water or more. The goal is to record ten stars per day. At the bottom of the page, you may want to jot down any thoughts or feelings regarding hunger, favorite meals, energy levels, moods, etc.

Day 7 of 21

Today's date: ____/____/____

BREAKFAST: Record your meal and give yourself a star for a Fat Flush Formula meal and if you drank 8 or more ounces of water.

Fat Flush meal star ⭐ 8 ounces of water star ⭐ Stars = ⭐

LUNCH: Record your meal and give yourself a star for a Fat Flush Formula meal and if you drank 8 or more ounces of water.

Fat Flush meal star ⭐ 8 ounces of water star ⭐ Stars = ⭐

SNACK: Record your meal and give yourself a star for a Fat Flush Formula meal and if you drank 8 or more ounces of water.

Fat Flush meal star ⭐ 8 ounces of water star ⭐ Stars = ⭐

DINNER: Record your meal and give yourself a star for a Fat Flush Formula meal and if you drank 8 or more ounces of water.

Fat Flush meal star ⭐ 8 ounces of water star ⭐ Stars = ⭐

EXERCISE: Describe your workout and give yourself a star for exercising and if you had 8 ounces or more of water.

Exercised ⭐ 8 ounces of water star ⭐ Stars = ⭐

NOTES: Record the total stars you achieved for the day, how you felt, and any notes:

TODAY'S TOTAL STARS = ⭐

Good job and congratulations, you're a STAR!

_____

(Your name)

21 DAY FAT FLUSH STAR TRACKER

This convenient 21-Day Fat Flush Star Tracker is a nutrition journal to help keep you motivated and assist you in reaching your goals. For the next 21 days, give yourself a star for each Fat Flush Formula meal you eat and jot down a brief description of the meal. Give yourself another star every time you drink 8 ounces of water or more. The goal is to record ten stars per day. At the bottom of the page, you may want to jot down any thoughts or feelings regarding hunger, favorite meals, energy levels, moods, etc.

Day 8 of 21

Today's date: ____/____/____

BREAKFAST: Record your meal and give yourself a star for a Fat Flush Formula meal and if you drank 8 or more ounces of water.

Fat Flush meal star ⭐ 8 ounces of water star ⭐ Stars = ⭐

LUNCH: Record your meal and give yourself a star for a Fat Flush Formula meal and if you drank 8 or more ounces of water.

Fat Flush meal star ⭐ 8 ounces of water star ⭐ Stars = ⭐

SNACK: Record your meal and give yourself a star for a Fat Flush Formula meal and if you drank 8 or more ounces of water.

Fat Flush meal star ⭐ 8 ounces of water star ⭐ Stars = ⭐

DINNER: Record your meal and give yourself a star for a Fat Flush Formula meal and if you drank 8 or more ounces of water.

Fat Flush meal star ⭐ 8 ounces of water star ⭐ Stars = ⭐

EXERCISE: Describe your workout and give yourself a star for exercising and if you had 8 ounces or more of water.

Exercised ⭐ 8 ounces of water star ⭐ Stars = ⭐

NOTES: Record the total stars you achieved for the day, how you felt, and any notes:

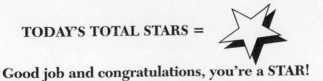

TODAY'S TOTAL STARS =

Good job and congratulations, you're a STAR!

_____

21 DAY FAT FLUSH STAR TRACKER

This convenient 21-Day Fat Flush Star Tracker is a nutrition journal to help keep you motivated and assist you in reaching your goals. For the next 21 days, give yourself a star for each Fat Flush Formula meal you eat and jot down a brief description of the meal. Give yourself another star every time you drink 8 ounces of water or more. The goal is to record ten stars per day. At the bottom of the page, you may want to jot down any thoughts or feelings regarding hunger, favorite meals, energy levels, moods, etc.

Day 9 of 21

Today's date: _____/_____/_____

BREAKFAST: Record your meal and give yourself a star for a Fat Flush Formula meal and if you drank 8 or more ounces of water.

Fat Flush meal star ⭐ 8 ounces of water star ⭐ Stars = ⭐

LUNCH: Record your meal and give yourself a star for a Fat Flush Formula meal and if you drank 8 or more ounces of water.

Fat Flush meal star ⭐ 8 ounces of water star ⭐ Stars = ⭐

SNACK: Record your meal and give yourself a star for a Fat Flush Formula meal and if you drank 8 or more ounces of water.

Fat Flush meal star ⭐ 8 ounces of water star ⭐ Stars = ⭐

DINNER: Record your meal and give yourself a star for a Fat Flush Formula meal and if you drank 8 or more ounces of water.

Fat Flush meal star ⭐ 8 ounces of water star ⭐ Stars = ⭐

EXERCISE: Describe your workout and give yourself a star for exercising and if you had 8 ounces or more of water.

Exercised ⭐ 8 ounces of water star ⭐ Stars = ⭐

NOTES: Record the total stars you achieved for the day, how you felt, and any notes:

TODAY'S TOTAL STARS = ⭐

Good job and congratulations, you're a STAR!

_____

(Your name)

21 DAY FAT FLUSH STAR TRACKER

This convenient 21-Day Fat Flush Star Tracker is a nutrition journal to help keep you motivated and assist you in reaching your goals. For the next 21 days, give yourself a star for each Fat Flush Formula meal you eat and jot down a brief description of the meal. Give yourself another star every time you drink 8 ounces of water or more. The goal is to record ten stars per day. At the bottom of the page, you may want to jot down any thoughts or feelings regarding hunger, favorite meals, energy levels, moods, etc.

Day 10 of 21

Today's date: _____/_____/_____

BREAKFAST: Record your meal and give yourself a star for a Fat Flush Formula meal and if you drank 8 or more ounces of water.

Fat Flush meal star ☆ 8 ounces of water star ☆ Stars = ☆

LUNCH: Record your meal and give yourself a star for a Fat Flush Formula meal and if you drank 8 or more ounces of water.

Fat Flush meal star ☆ 8 ounces of water star ☆ Stars = ☆

SNACK: Record your meal and give yourself a star for a Fat Flush Formula meal and if you drank 8 or more ounces of water.

Fat Flush meal star ☆ 8 ounces of water star ☆ Stars = ☆

DINNER: Record your meal and give yourself a star for a Fat Flush Formula meal and if you drank 8 or more ounces of water.

Fat Flush meal star ☆ 8 ounces of water star ☆ Stars = ☆

EXERCISE: Describe your workout and give yourself a star for exercising and if you had 8 ounces or more of water.

Exercised ☆ 8 ounces of water star ☆ Stars = ☆

NOTES: Record the total stars you achieved for the day, how you felt, and any notes:

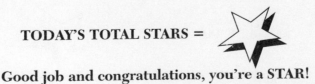

TODAY'S TOTAL STARS =

Good job and congratulations, you're a STAR!

_____
(Your name)

21 DAY FAT FLUSH STAR TRACKER

This convenient 21-Day Fat Flush Star Tracker is a nutrition journal to help keep you motivated and assist you in reaching your goals. For the next 21 days, give yourself a star for each Fat Flush Formula meal you eat and jot down a brief description of the meal. Give yourself another star every time you drink 8 ounces of water or more. The goal is to record ten stars per day. At the bottom of the page, you may want to jot down any thoughts or feelings regarding hunger, favorite meals, energy levels, moods, etc.

Day 11 of 21

Today's date: _____/_____/_____

BREAKFAST: Record your meal and give yourself a star for a Fat Flush Formula meal and if you drank 8 or more ounces of water.

Fat Flush meal star ⭐ 8 ounces of water star ⭐ Stars = ⭐

LUNCH: Record your meal and give yourself a star for a Fat Flush Formula meal and if you drank 8 or more ounces of water.

Fat Flush meal star ⭐ 8 ounces of water star ⭐ Stars = ⭐

SNACK: Record your meal and give yourself a star for a Fat Flush Formula meal and if you drank 8 or more ounces of water.

Fat Flush meal star ⭐ 8 ounces of water star ⭐ Stars = ⭐

DINNER: Record your meal and give yourself a star for a Fat Flush Formula meal and if you drank 8 or more ounces of water.

Fat Flush meal star ⭐ 8 ounces of water star ⭐ Stars = ⭐

EXERCISE: Describe your workout and give yourself a star for exercising and if you had 8 ounces or more of water.

Exercised ⭐ 8 ounces of water star ⭐ Stars = ⭐

NOTES: Record the total stars you achieved for the day, how you felt, and any notes:

TODAY'S TOTAL STARS = ⭐

Good job and congratulations, you're a STAR!

_____

(Your name)

21 DAY FAT FLUSH STAR TRACKER

This convenient 21-Day Fat Flush Star Tracker is a nutrition journal to help keep you motivated and assist you in reaching your goals. For the next 21 days, give yourself a star for each Fat Flush Formula meal you eat and jot down a brief description of the meal. Give yourself another star every time you drink 8 ounces of water or more. The goal is to record ten stars per day. At the bottom of the page, you may want to jot down any thoughts or feelings regarding hunger, favorite meals, energy levels, moods, etc.

Day 12 of 21

Today's date: _____/_____/_____

BREAKFAST: Record your meal and give yourself a star for a Fat Flush Formula meal and if you drank 8 or more ounces of water.

Fat Flush meal star ⭐   8 ounces of water star ⭐   Stars = ⭐

LUNCH: Record your meal and give yourself a star for a Fat Flush Formula meal and if you drank 8 or more ounces of water.

Fat Flush meal star ⭐   8 ounces of water star ⭐   Stars = ⭐

SNACK: Record your meal and give yourself a star for a Fat Flush Formula meal and if you drank 8 or more ounces of water.

Fat Flush meal star ⭐   8 ounces of water star ⭐   Stars = ⭐

DINNER: Record your meal and give yourself a star for a Fat Flush Formula meal and if you drank 8 or more ounces of water.

Fat Flush meal star ⭐   8 ounces of water star ⭐   Stars = ⭐

EXERCISE: Describe your workout and give yourself a star for exercising and if you had 8 ounces or more of water.

Exercised ⭐   8 ounces of water star ⭐   Stars = ⭐

NOTES: Record the total stars you achieved for the day, how you felt, and any notes:

TODAY'S TOTAL STARS = ⭐

Good job and congratulations, you're a STAR!

_____

(Your name)

21 DAY FAT FLUSH STAR TRACKER

This convenient 21-Day Fat Flush Star Tracker is a nutrition journal to help keep you motivated and assist you in reaching your goals. For the next 21 days, give yourself a star for each Fat Flush Formula meal you eat and jot down a brief description of the meal. Give yourself another star every time you drink 8 ounces of water or more. The goal is to record ten stars per day. At the bottom of the page, you may want to jot down any thoughts or feelings regarding hunger, favorite meals, energy levels, moods, etc.

Day 13 of 21
Today's date: ____/____/____

BREAKFAST: Record your meal and give yourself a star for a Fat Flush Formula meal and if you drank 8 or more ounces of water.

Fat Flush meal star ⭐ 8 ounces of water star ⭐ Stars = ⭐

LUNCH: Record your meal and give yourself a star for a Fat Flush Formula meal and if you drank 8 or more ounces of water.

Fat Flush meal star ⭐ 8 ounces of water star ⭐ Stars = ⭐

SNACK: Record your meal and give yourself a star for a Fat Flush Formula meal and if you drank 8 or more ounces of water.

Fat Flush meal star ⭐ 8 ounces of water star ⭐ Stars = ⭐

DINNER: Record your meal and give yourself a star for a Fat Flush Formula meal and if you drank 8 or more ounces of water.

Fat Flush meal star ⭐ 8 ounces of water star ⭐ Stars = ⭐

EXERCISE: Describe your workout and give yourself a star for exercising and if you had 8 ounces or more of water.

Exercised ⭐ 8 ounces of water star ⭐ Stars = ⭐

NOTES: Record the total stars you achieved for the day, how you felt, and any notes:

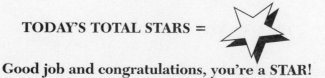

TODAY'S TOTAL STARS = ⭐

Good job and congratulations, you're a STAR!

_____
(Your name)

21 DAY FAT FLUSH STAR TRACKER

This convenient 21-Day Fat Flush Star Tracker is a nutrition journal to help keep you motivated and assist you in reaching your goals. For the next 21 days, give yourself a star for each Fat Flush Formula meal you eat and jot down a brief description of the meal. Give yourself another star every time you drink 8 ounces of water or more. The goal is to record ten stars per day. At the bottom of the page, you may want to jot down any thoughts or feelings regarding hunger, favorite meals, energy levels, moods, etc.

Day 14 of 21

Today's date: ____ / ____ / ____

BREAKFAST: Record your meal and give yourself a star for a Fat Flush Formula meal and if you drank 8 or more ounces of water.

Fat Flush meal star ⭐ 8 ounces of water star ⭐ Stars = ⭐

LUNCH: Record your meal and give yourself a star for a Fat Flush Formula meal and if you drank 8 or more ounces of water.

Fat Flush meal star ⭐ 8 ounces of water star ⭐ Stars = ⭐

SNACK: Record your meal and give yourself a star for a Fat Flush Formula meal and if you drank 8 or more ounces of water.

Fat Flush meal star ⭐ 8 ounces of water star ⭐ Stars = ⭐

DINNER: Record your meal and give yourself a star for a Fat Flush Formula meal and if you drank 8 or more ounces of water.

Fat Flush meal star ⭐ 8 ounces of water star ⭐ Stars = ⭐

EXERCISE: Describe your workout and give yourself a star for exercising and if you had 8 ounces or more of water.

Exercised ⭐ 8 ounces of water star ⭐ Stars = ⭐

NOTES: Record the total stars you achieved for the day, how you felt, and any notes:

TODAY'S TOTAL STARS = ⭐

Good job and congratulations, you're a STAR!

_____
(Your name)

21 DAY FAT FLUSH STAR TRACKER

This convenient 21-Day Fat Flush Star Tracker is a nutrition journal to help keep you motivated and assist you in reaching your goals. For the next 21 days, give yourself a star for each Fat Flush Formula meal you eat and jot down a brief description of the meal. Give yourself another star every time you drink 8 ounces of water or more. The goal is to record ten stars per day. At the bottom of the page, you may want to jot down any thoughts or feelings regarding hunger, favorite meals, energy levels, moods, etc.

Day 15 of 21

Today's date: _____/_____/_____

BREAKFAST: Record your meal and give yourself a star for a Fat Flush Formula meal and if you drank 8 or more ounces of water.

Fat Flush meal star ⭐ 8 ounces of water star ⭐ Stars = ⭐

LUNCH: Record your meal and give yourself a star for a Fat Flush Formula meal and if you drank 8 or more ounces of water.

Fat Flush meal star ⭐ 8 ounces of water star ⭐ Stars = ⭐

SNACK: Record your meal and give yourself a star for a Fat Flush Formula meal and if you drank 8 or more ounces of water.

Fat Flush meal star ⭐ 8 ounces of water star ⭐ Stars = ⭐

DINNER: Record your meal and give yourself a star for a Fat Flush Formula meal and if you drank 8 or more ounces of water.

Fat Flush meal star ⭐ 8 ounces of water star ⭐ Stars = ⭐

EXERCISE: Describe your workout and give yourself a star for exercising and if you had 8 ounces or more of water.

Exercised ⭐ 8 ounces of water star ⭐ Stars = ⭐

NOTES: Record the total stars you achieved for the day, how you felt, and any notes:

TODAY'S TOTAL STARS = ⭐

Good job and congratulations, you're a STAR!

_____
(Your name)

21 DAY FAT FLUSH STAR TRACKER

This convenient 21-Day Fat Flush Star Tracker is a nutrition journal to help keep you motivated and assist you in reaching your goals. For the next 21 days, give yourself a star for each Fat Flush Formula meal you eat and jot down a brief description of the meal. Give yourself another star every time you drink 8 ounces of water or more. The goal is to record ten stars per day. At the bottom of the page, you may want to jot down any thoughts or feelings regarding hunger, favorite meals, energy levels, moods, etc.

Day 16 of 21

Today's date: _____/_____/_____

BREAKFAST: Record your meal and give yourself a star for a Fat Flush Formula meal and if you drank 8 or more ounces of water.

Fat Flush meal star ⭐ 8 ounces of water star ⭐ Stars = ⭐

LUNCH: Record your meal and give yourself a star for a Fat Flush Formula meal and if you drank 8 or more ounces of water.

Fat Flush meal star ⭐ 8 ounces of water star ⭐ Stars = ⭐

SNACK: Record your meal and give yourself a star for a Fat Flush Formula meal and if you drank 8 or more ounces of water.

Fat Flush meal star ⭐ 8 ounces of water star ⭐ Stars = ⭐

DINNER: Record your meal and give yourself a star for a Fat Flush Formula meal and if you drank 8 or more ounces of water.

Fat Flush meal star ⭐ 8 ounces of water star ⭐ Stars = ⭐

EXERCISE: Describe your workout and give yourself a star for exercising and if you had 8 ounces or more of water.

Exercised ⭐ 8 ounces of water star ⭐ Stars = ⭐

NOTES: Record the total stars you achieved for the day, how you felt, and any notes:

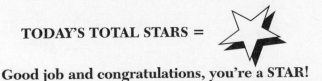

TODAY'S TOTAL STARS =

Good job and congratulations, you're a STAR!

_____
(Your name)

21 DAY FAT FLUSH STAR TRACKER

This convenient 21-Day Fat Flush Star Tracker is a nutrition journal to help keep you motivated and assist you in reaching your goals. For the next 21 days, give yourself a star for each Fat Flush Formula meal you eat and jot down a brief description of the meal. Give yourself another star every time you drink 8 ounces of water or more. The goal is to record ten stars per day. At the bottom of the page, you may want to jot down any thoughts or feelings regarding hunger, favorite meals, energy levels, moods, etc.

Day 17 of 21
Today's date: ____/____/____

BREAKFAST: Record your meal and give yourself a star for a Fat Flush Formula meal and if you drank 8 or more ounces of water.

Fat Flush meal star ⭐ 8 ounces of water star ⭐ Stars = ⭐

LUNCH: Record your meal and give yourself a star for a Fat Flush Formula meal and if you drank 8 or more ounces of water.

Fat Flush meal star ⭐ 8 ounces of water star ⭐ Stars = ⭐

SNACK: Record your meal and give yourself a star for a Fat Flush Formula meal and if you drank 8 or more ounces of water.

Fat Flush meal star ⭐ 8 ounces of water star ⭐ Stars = ⭐

DINNER: Record your meal and give yourself a star for a Fat Flush Formula meal and if you drank 8 or more ounces of water.

Fat Flush meal star ⭐ 8 ounces of water star ⭐ Stars = ⭐

EXERCISE: Describe your workout and give yourself a star for exercising and if you had 8 ounces or more of water.

Exercised ⭐ 8 ounces of water star ⭐ Stars = ⭐

NOTES: Record the total stars you achieved for the day, how you felt, and any notes:

TODAY'S TOTAL STARS = ⭐

Good job and congratulations, you're a STAR!

21 DAY FAT FLUSH STAR TRACKER

This convenient 21-Day Fat Flush Star Tracker is a nutrition journal to help keep you motivated and assist you in reaching your goals. For the next 21 days, give yourself a star for each Fat Flush Formula meal you eat and jot down a brief description of the meal. Give yourself another star every time you drink 8 ounces of water or more. The goal is to record ten stars per day. At the bottom of the page, you may want to jot down any thoughts or feelings regarding hunger, favorite meals, energy levels, moods, etc.

Day 18 of 21
Today's date: ____/____/____

BREAKFAST: Record your meal and give yourself a star for a Fat Flush Formula meal and if you drank 8 or more ounces of water.

Fat Flush meal star ⭐ 8 ounces of water star ⭐ Stars = ⭐

LUNCH: Record your meal and give yourself a star for a Fat Flush Formula meal and if you drank 8 or more ounces of water.

Fat Flush meal star ⭐ 8 ounces of water star ⭐ Stars = ⭐

SNACK: Record your meal and give yourself a star for a Fat Flush Formula meal and if you drank 8 or more ounces of water.

Fat Flush meal star ⭐ 8 ounces of water star ⭐ Stars = ⭐

DINNER: Record your meal and give yourself a star for a Fat Flush Formula meal and if you drank 8 or more ounces of water.

Fat Flush meal star ⭐ 8 ounces of water star ⭐ Stars = ⭐

EXERCISE: Describe your workout and give yourself a star for exercising and if you had 8 ounces or more of water.

Exercised ⭐ 8 ounces of water star ⭐ Stars = ⭐

NOTES: Record the total stars you achieved for the day, how you felt, and any notes:

TODAY'S TOTAL STARS = ⭐

Good job and congratulations, you're a STAR!

_____
(Your name)

21 DAY FAT FLUSH STAR TRACKER

This convenient 21-Day Fat Flush Star Tracker is a nutrition journal to help keep you motivated and assist you in reaching your goals. For the next 21 days, give yourself a star for each Fat Flush Formula meal you eat and jot down a brief description of the meal. Give yourself another star every time you drink 8 ounces of water or more. The goal is to record ten stars per day. At the bottom of the page, you may want to jot down any thoughts or feelings regarding hunger, favorite meals, energy levels, moods, etc.

Day 19 of 21
Today's date: ____/____/____

BREAKFAST: Record your meal and give yourself a star for a Fat Flush Formula meal and if you drank 8 or more ounces of water.

Fat Flush meal star ⭐ 8 ounces of water star ⭐ Stars = ⭐

LUNCH: Record your meal and give yourself a star for a Fat Flush Formula meal and if you drank 8 or more ounces of water.

Fat Flush meal star ⭐ 8 ounces of water star ⭐ Stars = ⭐

SNACK: Record your meal and give yourself a star for a Fat Flush Formula meal and if you drank 8 or more ounces of water.

Fat Flush meal star ⭐ 8 ounces of water star ⭐ Stars = ⭐

DINNER: Record your meal and give yourself a star for a Fat Flush Formula meal and if you drank 8 or more ounces of water.

Fat Flush meal star ⭐ 8 ounces of water star ⭐ Stars = ⭐

EXERCISE: Describe your workout and give yourself a star for exercising and if you had 8 ounces or more of water.

Exercised ⭐ 8 ounces of water star ⭐ Stars = ⭐

NOTES: Record the total stars you achieved for the day, how you felt, and any notes:

TODAY'S TOTAL STARS = ⭐

Good job and congratulations, you're a STAR!

(Your name)

21 DAY FAT FLUSH STAR TRACKER

This convenient 21-Day Fat Flush Star Tracker is a nutrition journal to help keep you motivated and assist you in reaching your goals. For the next 21 days, give yourself a star for each Fat Flush Formula meal you eat and jot down a brief description of the meal. Give yourself another star every time you drink 8 ounces of water or more. The goal is to record ten stars per day. At the bottom of the page, you may want to jot down any thoughts or feelings regarding hunger, favorite meals, energy levels, moods, etc.

Day 20 of 21

Today's date: _____/_____/_____

BREAKFAST: Record your meal and give yourself a star for a Fat Flush Formula meal and if you drank 8 or more ounces of water.

Fat Flush meal star ⭐ 8 ounces of water star ⭐ Stars = ⭐

LUNCH: Record your meal and give yourself a star for a Fat Flush Formula meal and if you drank 8 or more ounces of water.

Fat Flush meal star ⭐ 8 ounces of water star ⭐ Stars = ⭐

SNACK: Record your meal and give yourself a star for a Fat Flush Formula meal and if you drank 8 or more ounces of water.

Fat Flush meal star ⭐ 8 ounces of water star ⭐ Stars = ⭐

DINNER: Record your meal and give yourself a star for a Fat Flush Formula meal and if you drank 8 or more ounces of water.

Fat Flush meal star ⭐ 8 ounces of water star ⭐ Stars = ⭐

EXERCISE: Describe your workout and give yourself a star for exercising and if you had 8 ounces or more of water.

Exercised ⭐ 8 ounces of water star ⭐ Stars = ⭐

NOTES: Record the total stars you achieved for the day, how you felt, and any notes:

TODAY'S TOTAL STARS = ⭐

Good job and congratulations, you're a STAR!

21 DAY FAT FLUSH STAR TRACKER

This convenient 21-Day Fat Flush Star Tracker is a nutrition journal to help keep you motivated and assist you in reaching your goals. For the next 21 days, give yourself a star for each Fat Flush Formula meal you eat and jot down a brief description of the meal. Give yourself another star every time you drink 8 ounces of water or more. The goal is to record ten stars per day. At the bottom of the page, you may want to jot down any thoughts or feelings regarding hunger, favorite meals, energy levels, moods, etc.

Day 21 of 21

Today's date: _____/_____/_____

BREAKFAST: Record your meal and give yourself a star for a Fat Flush Formula meal and if you drank 8 or more ounces of water.

Fat Flush meal star ⭐ 8 ounces of water star ⭐ Stars = ⭐

LUNCH: Record your meal and give yourself a star for a Fat Flush Formula meal and if you drank 8 or more ounces of water.

Fat Flush meal star ⭐ 8 ounces of water star ⭐ Stars = ⭐

SNACK: Record your meal and give yourself a star for a Fat Flush Formula meal and if you drank 8 or more ounces of water.

Fat Flush meal star ⭐ 8 ounces of water star ⭐ Stars = ⭐

DINNER: Record your meal and give yourself a star for a Fat Flush Formula meal and if you drank 8 or more ounces of water.

Fat Flush meal star ⭐ 8 ounces of water star ⭐ Stars = ⭐

EXERCISE: Describe your workout and give yourself a star for exercising and if you had 8 ounces or more of water.

Exercised ⭐ 8 ounces of water star ⭐ Stars = ⭐

NOTES: Record the total stars you achieved for the day, how you felt, and any notes:

TODAY'S TOTAL STARS = ⭐

Good job and congratulations, you're a STAR!

_____
(Your name)

FORMULA FOR LIFE MONTHLY TRACKER

Use this guide to help you keep track of all the great results you can achieve when following the Formula for Life 40-30-30 nutrition program. Once a month, fill in the blanks with your results.

Month 1: Date: _____ Weight: _____ % Body Fat: _____ Pant/Dress size: _____
Others: _____

Month 2: Date: _____ Weight: _____ % Body Fat: _____ Pant/Dress size: _____
Others: _____

Month 3: Date: _____ Weight: _____ % Body Fat: _____ Pant/Dress size: _____
Others: _____

Month 4: Date: _____ Weight: _____ % Body Fat: _____ Pant/Dress size: _____
Others: _____

Month 5: Date: _____ Weight: _____ % Body Fat: _____ Pant/Dress size: _____
Others: _____

Month 6: Date: _____ Weight: _____ % Body Fat: _____ Pant/Dress size: _____
Others: _____

Month 7: Date: _____ Weight: _____ % Body Fat: _____ Pant/Dress size: _____
Others: _____

Month 8: Date: _____ Weight: _____ % Body Fat: _____ Pant/Dress size: _____
Others: _____

Month 9: Date: _____ Weight: _____ % Body Fat: _____ Pant/Dress size: _____
Others: _____

Month 10: Date: _____ Weight: _____ % Body Fat: _____ Pant/Dress size: _____
Others: _____

Month 11: Date: _____ Weight: _____ % Body Fat: _____ Pant/Dress size: _____
Others: _____

Month 12: Date: _____ Weight: _____ % Body Fat: _____ Pant/Dress size: _____
Others: _____

Chapter Twenty-six

HOW TO MAKE A
40-30-30 MEAL

Through the years, we have found that the easiest way for you to learn how to make your own 40-30-30 Formula meals is to begin by following the personalized meal plans we have provided. By using these meals, you can get a better idea of what a 40-30-30 Formula meal should look like. When you begin to design your own meals, there are four easy steps to follow:

1. Review the Formula Meal Plan Selection Chart for the meal plan that is right for you.

2. Use the Macronutrient Chart on page 276 to determine how much carbohydrate, protein, and fat you need at each meal.

3. Choose from foods listed in the Quick Reference Food Value and Glycemic Index Guide or from any other source.

4. Use the Design Your Own Formula Meal Worksheet to help design your own 40-30-30 Formula meals. Make sure the carbohydrate, protein, and fat grams are close to your requirements.

DESIGN YOUR OWN
FAT FLUSH FORMULA MEALS

Step 1.

40% Carbohydrate—Use only low to medium glycemic fruits and vegetables.

Step 2.

30% Protein—Choose high quality, lowfat protein at each meal.

Step 3.

30% Fat—Have one serving of good fat at each meal.

DESIGN YOUR OWN
REGULAR FORMULA MEALS

Step 1.

40% Carbohydrate—Have one serving of high glycemic carbohydrate and the rest from low to medium glycemic rated fruits and vegetables.

Step 2.

30% Protein—Choose high quality, lowfat protein at each meal.

Step 3.

30% Fat—Have one serving of good fat at each meal.

EASY SUBSTITUTIONS

Carbohydrate Substitutions—You can substitute any vegetable for any other vegetable, any fruit for any other fruit, and any starch for any other starch as long as they are rated about the same on the glycemic index.

Protein Substitutions—You can substitute any lowfat protein for any other lowfat protein. Vegetarians should substitute any unacceptable protein with equal amounts of lowfat vegetarian protein that is low in carbohydrates and fat, such as lowfat tofu or tempeh.

Fat Substitutions—You can substitute any oil for any other oil, any nut for any other nut, or any lowfat cheese for any other cheese. You can also substitute full fat mayonnaise for avocado.

DESIGN YOUR OWN
FORMULA MEAL WORKSHEET

(Use as an original and make photocopies of this worksheet)

Food	Carb. Grams	Protein Grams	Fat Grams
_____	_____	_____	_____
_____	_____	_____	_____
_____	_____	_____	_____
_____	_____	_____	_____
_____	_____	_____	_____
_____	_____	_____	_____
_____	_____	_____	_____
_____	_____	_____	_____
_____	_____	_____	_____
_____	_____	_____	_____
_____	_____	_____	_____
TOTALS	_____	_____	_____

THE FORMULA
MEAL PLAN SELECTION CHART

WOMEN

Activity Level	Low–Moderate	Medium–High
Hours of Exercise per Week	Exercise 0–4 hours per week	Exercise 5–10 hours per week
Current Body Weight	*Use Meal Planner*	*Use Meal Planner*
Under 140	A	B
141–180	B	C
181–200+	C	D

MEN

Activity Level	Low–Moderate	Medium–High
Hours of Exercise per Week	Exercise 0–4 hours per week	Exercise 5–10 hours per week
Current Body Weight	*Use Meal Planner*	*Use Meal Planner*
Under 140	B	C
141–180	C	D
181–250+	C	D

Your Personalized Meal Plan is _____

THE FORMULA
MEAL PLAN SELECTION CHART FOR ELITE ATHLETES

FEMALE ELITE ATHLETES

Current Body Weight	Train 10 or more hours per week
Under 140	C
141–180	D
180 and over	E

MALE ELITE ATHLETES

Current Body Weight	Train 10 or more hours per week
Under 140	C
141–180	D
180 and over	E

MACRONUTRIENT CHART

Listed below you will find the total grams of carbohydrate, protein, fat, and calories listed for each meal plan. The meal plans have been tailored for individual requirements based on gender, weight, and activity levels. To determine which meal plan is right for you, refer to the Formula Meal Plan Selection Chart. Each meal and snack contains the 40-30-30 ratio, which provides 40 percent of its *total calories* from carbohydrates, 30 percent from protein, and 30 percent from fat.

Personal Meal Plan	A	B	C	D	E
BREAKFAST					
Carbohydrate grams	20	20	33	47	53
Protein grams	15	15	25	35	40
Fat grams	6	6	11	13	18
Calories	194	194	331	445	534
LUNCH					
Carbohydrate grams	27	40	40	53	66
Protein grams	20	30	30	40	50
Fat grams	9	14	14	18	22
Calories	269	406	406	534	662
SNACKS					
Carbohydrate grams	20	20	20	20	40
Protein grams	15	15	15	15	30
Fat grams	6	6	6	6	12
Calories	194	194	194	194	388
DINNER					
Carbohydrate grams	40	47	53	53	66
Protein grams	30	35	40	40	50
Fat grams	14	15	18	18	22
Calories	406	463	534	534	662

Personal Meal Plan	A	B	C	D	E
DAILY TOTALS					
Carbohydrate grams	106	126	146	173	226
Protein grams	80	95	110	130	170
Fat grams	35	42	48	57	75
Calories	1063	1257	1465	1707	2246

QUICK REFERENCE
FOOD VALUE AND GLYCEMIC INDEX GUIDE

The chart below includes the carbohydrate, protein, and fat breakdown for one serving of each food and the approximate glycemic index rating for carbohydrate foods. The glycemic index indicates how quickly a food can elevate blood sugar. Note: Foods can vary by brand names, so always refer to the actual Nutrition Facts panel when available for the most accurate numbers.

Glycemic Index ratings: L = low (0–39 rating), M = medium (40–75 rating), H = high (76–112 rating), and VH = very high (113–150 rating). The ratings are based on white bread = 100.

CARBOHYDRATE SOURCES

Food	Serving Size	Glycemic Rating	Carb. Grams	Protein Grams	Fat Grams
FRUITS					
Apple	1 medium	M	21	0	0
Applesauce (unsweetened)	½ cup	M	25	0	0
Banana	1 each	H	28	1	1
Blueberries, raw	½ cup	L	10	1	0
Cantaloupe	½ melon	M	23	2	1
Cherries	½ cup	L	9	1	0

Food	Serving Size	Glycemic Rating	Carb. Grams	Protein Grams	Fat Grams
Grapefruit	½ fruit	L	10	1	0
Grapes	10 fruits	M	4	0	0
Kiwifruit	1 medium	L	11	1	0
Mango, cubed	½ cup	H	14	1	0
Orange	1 fruit	M	15	1	0
Papaya, cubed	½ cup	M	7	0	0
Peach, fresh, 2½-inch	1 fruit	M	11	1	0
Peaches, canned/water	½ cup	M	7	1	0
Pear, fresh, 2½-inch	1 fruit	M	25	1	0
Pears, canned/water	½ cup	M	10	0	0
Pineapple, fresh	1 cup	H	19	1	1
Plum, raw, 2⅛-inch	1 fruit	L	9	1	0
Strawberries	1 cup	L	10	1	0
Tangerine	1 fruit	M	9	1	0
Watermelon, cubed	1 cup	H	11	1	0
Fruit cocktail, canned, in water	1 cup	M	20	1	0
Raisins	¼ cup	H	29	1	0
Dates	1 fruit	VH	6	0	0

VEGETABLES

Food	Serving Size	Glycemic Rating	Carb. Grams	Protein Grams	Fat Grams
Artichoke, cooked	1 medium	L	13	4	0
Asparagus	1 cup	L	6	3	0
Bok choy	½ cup	L	1	0	0
Broccoli	1 cup	L	4	2	0
Butternut squash	½ cup	M	8	1	0
Brussels sprouts	1 cup	L	8	3	1
Cabbage, shredded	1 cup	L	5	1	0
Carrots, cooked	1 cup	H	13	1	0
Cauliflower	1 cup	L	5	2	0
Celery, raw	1 stalk	L	1	0	0

Food	Serving Size	Glycemic Rating	Carb. Grams	Protein Grams	Fat Grams
Cucumber, sliced	½ cup	L	1	0	0
Corn, kernels	½ cup	H	15	2	1
Corn on the cob	½ ear	H	9	1	1
Green beans (snap)	1 cup	L	8	2	0
Green pepper	½ cup	L	5	1	0
Lentils, cooked	½ cup	M	20	9	0
Lettuce					
Iceberg	1 cup	L	1	1	0
Butterhead	5 leaves	L	1	0	0
Romaine	1 cup	L	1	1	0
Mushrooms, raw	½ cup	L	2	1	0
Peas, green, cooked	½ cup	M	10	4	0
Salsa	1 oz.	L	2	0	0
Snow peas, raw	½ cup	L	2	1	0
Spinach, raw	½ cup	L	1	1	0
Spinach, boiled, drained	½ cup	L	3	3	0
Summer squash, boiled	½ cup	M	2	1	0
Tomato	1 medium	L	6	1	0
Tomato sauce (no sugar)	½ cup	L	9	2	0
Zucchini, raw	½ cup	L	2	1	0

BREADS/STARCHES

Food	Serving Size	Glycemic Rating	Carb. Grams	Protein Grams	Fat Grams
Bagel, plain	1 each	H	48	9	1
Barley, cooked	½ cup	M	22	2	0
Bread					
white	1 slice	H	12	2	1
wheat	1 slice	H	12	3	1
reduced calorie	1 slice	H	10	0	0
rye (pumpernickel)	1 slice	H	15	3	1
French	1 slice	VH	13	2	1

Food	Serving Size	Glycemic Rating	Carb. Grams	Protein Grams	Fat Grams
Buns					
hamburger or hot dog	1 each	H	22	4	2
reduced calorie	1 each	H	18	4	1
English muffin	1 each	H	26	4	1
Pita bread, 6.5-inch diameter	1 each	H	33	5	1
Kashi, cooked	½ cup	M	30	6	3
Muffins, bran	1 medium	H	24	4	6
Oatmeal, cooked	1 cup	M	24	6	2
Pancakes, 4 inches each	1 each	H	14	2	1
Pasta, cooked	1 cup	M	63	11	1
Popcorn, air popped	3 cup	VH	19	3	1
Potato, baked	1 medium	VH	22	3	0
Potato, mashed	½ cup	VH	14	2	2
Potato, red, new	½ cup	M	13	2	0
Rice, brown, cooked	1 cup	H	46	5	2
Rice, white, cooked	1 cup	H	52	5	1
Sweet potato, medium	½ each	H	16	1	0
Tortilla, corn, 7-inch diameter	1 item	M	12	1	1
Tortilla, flour, 9-inch diameter	1 item	H	22	3	4
Waffles, 4-inch square	1 item	H	14	2	3
Yam, cooked	½ cup	H	21	1	0
Beans					
Baked beans, canned	½ cup	M	26	6	1
Kidney beans, canned	½ cup	M	19	7	0
Pinto beans, canned	½ cup	M	17	5	0

PROTEIN SOURCES

Food	Serving Size	Carb. Grams	Protein Grams	Fat Grams
BEEF				
Deli-sliced roast beef	4 oz.	0	37	9
Lean flank steak	4 oz.	0	31	11
Ground sirloin, extra lean	4 oz.	0	30	9
Tenderloin	4 oz.	0	32	12
CHICKEN				
Chicken breast, w/o skin	4 oz.	0	25	3
Deli-sliced chicken breast	4 oz.	0	25	3
DAIRY				
American cheese, lite	1 oz.	3	5	4
American cheese, fat free	1 oz.	1	8	0
Mozzarella, lite	1 oz.	1	9	2
Mozzarella, fat free	1 oz.	1	9	0
Parmesan, grated, lite	1 oz.	1	15	4
Ricotta, lite	1 oz.	1	4	2
String cheese, lite	1 oz.	1	9	2
Cottage cheese, 2%	1 cup	8	31	4
Cottage cheese, 1%	1 cup	6	28	2
Cottage cheese, nonfat	1 cup	6	29	0
Cottage cheese, dry curd	½ cup	3	25	1
Cream cheese, nonfat	1 oz.	2	4	0
Milk, 2% lowfat	8 oz.	11	8	4
Milk, 1% lowfat	8 oz.	11	7	2
Milk, nonfat	8 oz.	11	8	0
Sour cream, nonfat	2 tbsp.	3	2	0
Yogurt, plain, fat free	8 oz.	17	13	0
Yogurt, plain, lowfat	8 oz.	16	12	4

Food	Serving Size	Carb. Grams	Protein Grams	Fat Grams
EGGS				
Egg, large	one	1	5	4
Egg white	one	0	4	0
Egg substitute	¼ cup	1	6	0
LAMB				
Chop, lean only	4 oz.	0	25	9
PORK				
Ham, deli-sliced	4 oz.	1	22	6
Pork tenderloin, roasted	4 oz.	0	24	4
PROTEIN POWDER				
Pure whey protein powder	1 scoop (22.2 grams)	0	20	0
SEAFOOD				
Flounder	6 oz.	0	32	2
Halibut	6 oz.	0	35	4
Lobster	6 oz.	1	35	1
Salmon, smoked	6 oz.	0	34	6
Salmon, coho	6 oz.	0	34	6
Scallops	6 oz.	4	28	1
Sea bass	6 oz.	0	31	3
Shrimp	6 oz.	0	35	2
Snapper	6 oz.	0	35	2
Sole	6 oz.	0	32	2
Swordfish	6 oz.	0	34	7
Rainbow trout	6 oz.	0	35	6
Tuna, albacore, canned (water)	6 oz.	0	43	1
Tuna, steak	6 oz.	0	40	8

Food	Serving Size	Carb. Grams	Protein Grams	Fat Grams
TURKEY				
Breast, w/o skin, roasted	4 oz.	0	28	1
Breast, w/o skin, ground	4 oz.	0	28	1
Premium sliced deli breast	4 oz.	0	25	2
TOFU				
Tofu, extra firm	4 oz.	3	9	5
Tofu, soft	4 oz.	3	5	3
Tempeh	1 oz.	5	5	2
VENISON				
Venison (meat only)	4 oz.	0	26	3

FAT SOURCES

Food	Serving Size	Carb. Grams	Protein Grams	Fat Grams
NUTS AND SEEDS				
Almonds, raw	1 tbsp.	2	2	5
Almond butter	1 tsp.	3	2	9
Peanuts	1 tbsp.	1	2	4
Peanut butter	1 tbsp.	3	4	8
Pistachios, raw	1 tbsp.	2	2	4
Pumpkin seeds, raw	1 tbsp.	2	2	4
Sesame seeds, raw	1 tbsp.	3	3	4
Sunflower seeds, raw	1 tbsp.	3	3	4
Walnuts, raw	1 tbsp.	1	2	4

Food	Serving Size	Carb. Grams	Protein Grams	Fat Grams
OILS AND SPREADS				
Avocado	¼ fruit	4	1	8
Butter	1 tbsp.	0	0	11
Cream Cheese, Philly Light	2 tbsp.	0	1	5
Flaxseed oil	1 tbsp.	0	0	14
Mayonnaise	1 tbsp.	0	0	14
Olive oil	1 tbsp.	0	0	14
Olives	5 medium	1	0	3
Olives, Greek style	5 medium	1	0	3
Peanut oil	1 tbsp.	0	0	14
Safflower oil	1 tbsp.	0	0	14
Sour cream, lite	1 tbsp.	2	1	1
Vegetable oil	1 tbsp.	0	0	14
Wheat germ oil	1 tbsp.	0	0	14

Chapter Twenty-seven

THE FORMULA SHOPPING GUIDE

Research has shown that dieters who follow precise meal plans and use a shopping list have better results than those who don't. With that in mind, we developed a convenient shopping guide for you to use to prepare your shopping list. Review either the Fat Flush Formula meals or the Regular Formula meals and choose a few from breakfast, lunch, snacks, and dinner that sound good to you.

CARBOHYDRATES

Fruits

apples	cherries, dried
applesauce	grapefruits
apricots	grapefruit sections with juice
blueberries, fresh or frozen	grapes
cantaloupes	kiwis
cherries	lemons

lemon juice

mixed berries, frozen

oranges

orange juice

peaches, fresh, frozen, or canned

pears, fresh or canned

pineapple, fresh or canned

plums

preserves, fruit

strawberries, fresh or frozen

tangerines

Vegetables

asparagus

bean sprouts

broccoli

cabbage, red or green

carrots

cauliflower

celery

cherry tomatoes

coleslaw, deli made

cucumber

eggplant

green beans, fresh or canned

green bell pepper

green onions

lettuce, iceberg

lettuce, red leaf

lettuce, romaine

mushrooms

onion, sweet

onions, white pearl

parsley

red bell pepper

snow peas

spinach

shallots

tomatoes, canned

tomatoes, fresh

tomato paste, canned

tomato sauce

zucchini

Starches

bran cereal

All-Bran cereal

bagel, plain, wheat, or oat bran

barley, pearl

black beans, canned

bran muffin, lowfat

bread

bread, reduced calorie

corn, canned

corn chips

corn on the cob

croutons

English muffin

French bread, loaf

garbanzo beans, canned

granola

hamburger bun

Italian bread crumbs

kidney beans, canned

lasagna noodles

macaroni, elbow

oatmeal

pasta

pinto beans, canned

pita bread

potatoes, little red

refried beans

rye crackers (Wasa)

rice, brown

rice, white

shredded wheat

taco shells

tortillas, corn, 5-inch

tortillas, flour, 7- to 8-inch

PROTEIN

Boca burger, fat free

beef, cubed, extra lean

Canadian bacon

Cheddar cheese, lowfat

chicken breast, deli-sliced

chicken breast, raw

chicken breast, precooked

cottage cheese

crabmeat

eggs

feta cheese, reduced fat

fish, white, cod

ground sirloin, extra lean

Gruyère cheese

ham, deli style

jalapeño cheese

Knudsen Cottage Doubles (four-pack)

Knudsen On the Go (four-pack cottage cheese)

Knudsen On the Go (four-pack cottage cheese and fruit)

lobster meat

lox

milk, nonfat

milk, 1% lowfat

mozzarella cheese

Parmesan cheese

pork tenderloin

red snapper

ricotta cheese, fat free

salmon steaks

sausage, chicken or turkey, lowfat

shrimp, cooked or raw

soybeans, raw

soy milk, lowfat, plain

string cheese, lowfat

Swiss cheese, lowfat

tempeh

tofu

tuna, albacore (water-packed)

tuna salad, deli style

turkey breast, ground

turkey breast, deli-sliced

turkey breast, whole

yogurt, plain, nonfat

yogurt, flavored

FAT

almonds, raw

almond butter

avocado

blue cheese, crumbled

butter, stick

butter, whipped

canola oil

coleslaw dressing

cream cheese, full fat

cream cheese, lowfat

Kalamata olives

macadamia nuts

mayonnaise, full fat

mayonnaise, lowfat

olive oil

olive oil spray

olives, black, large

peanut butter

peanut oil

pecans

pesto sauce

salad dressing, full fat

salad dressing, lowfat

sesame oil

sour cream, lowfat

sour cream, nonfat

sunflower seeds

vegetable oil

walnuts

MISCELLANEOUS ITEMS

allspice

anchovy paste (in tube)

barbecue sauce, bottled

basil

bay leaves

beef broth, canned

California rolls with tuna or salmon

catsup

cayenne pepper

chicken broth, canned

chili powder

chili seasoning, packaged

chili sauce

cilantro, fresh

cinnamon

cocktail sauce

cocoa powder, unsweetened

cornstarch

cumin

dill, fresh

dill pickles

dry cooking sherry

fructose, granulated

garlic cloves

green chili peppers, canned

ginger, ground

horseradish, prepared

honey

hot pepper sauce

Italian seasonings

meat marinade

Mexican seasonings

mustard, Dijon

mustard, dry

mustard, prepared

Nescafé Decaf French Roast
   instant coffee

oregano

paprika

pasta sauce, fat free

peanut sauce

pepper

pickle relish, sweet or dill

pizza sauce

red pepper flakes, dried

rosemary, dried

salsa

salt

soy sauce

taco seasoning, packaged

teriyaki marinade

thyme, dried

wine, red or white

Worcestershire sauce

vanilla

SUPPLEMENTS

40-30-30 Nutrition Bar

40-30-30 powdered drink mix

bee pollen

Emer'gen-C packets

flax oil

pure whey protein powder

(These items can typically be found
   in health food stores)

DESSERT RECIPES

THE FORMULA SHOPPING GUIDE

Review the Fat Flush Formula and the Regular Formula dessert recipes and choose your favorites to prepare your shopping list.

Carbohydrates

brown sugar

chocolate squares, semisweet, baking

cocoa powder (unsweetened)

coconut (flaked and sweetened)

flour

frozen yogurt, vanilla, lowfat

fructose, granulated

graham crackers, honey or chocolate

ice cream, vanilla, lowfat

oatmeal (rolled oats)

powdered sugar

pumpkin, canned

sugar

Proteins

cottage cheese, 2% lowfat

cream cheese, Philadelphia Brand Fat Free (8 oz. box)

cream cheese, Philadelphia Brand ⅓ Less Fat (8 oz. box)

cream cheese, Philadelphia Light Whipped (in plastic tub)

eggs, large

milk, nonfat

pure whey protein powder

sour cream, fatfree

tofu, lowfat, silken (comes in a box or tub)

Fats

almond butter (available in health food stores)

almonds (sliced)

butter

old-fashioned peanut butter (smooth or chunky)

walnuts

Flavorings and Miscellaneous

baking powder

cinnamon, ground

cloves, ground

cornstarch

ginger, ground

instant espresso coffee powder

lemon juice

nutmeg, ground

orange

orange extract

vanilla

Chapter Twenty-eight

SUPPLEMENT RESOURCE GUIDE

What about supplements? We are often asked about supplements. The bottom line is, to maximize your health and fat burning ability, you need to eat a healthy, balanced diet. No matter what type of supplement or how much you take, you will never get the results you are looking for until you first get your diet balanced.

There are a few 40-30-30 meal replacement bars and shakes that we recommend. They offer convenience and make life a little easier. They are not designed to permanently replace meals but can be used when it is inconvenient to make a 40-30-30 Formula meal. These 40-30-30 food supplements help make following the Formula so easy, anyone can do it. Listed below are a few of the supplements that we use and recommend.

40-30-30 NUTRITION BARS

These supplement bars make following the Formula even easier. They are the ultimate fast food. There are several companies that manufacture

40-30-30 Nutrition Bars. Many taste great and you can use them in place of a small meal or snack. So instead of skipping a meal, or when preparing a meal is inconvenient, you can eat a 40-30-30 Nutrition Bar. We have been using these bars since 1991 and love them. They are especially useful when you travel. They are also recommended before or after exercise.

A good nutrition bar should be balanced. For the best results, make sure your bar uses the 40-30-30 nutrition ratio. Listed below is an approximate nutritional profile for a 40-30-30 Nutrition Bar. Use this sample when shopping for a balanced nutrition bar:

NUTRITION BAR NUTRITIONAL PROFILE

Calories:	190–200
Carbohydrates:	20 grams
Protein:	14 grams
Fat:	6 grams

Below are several 40-30-30 Nutrition Bars that we use and recommend:

- Balance Bar by the Balance Bar Company
- 40-30-30 Bar by Trader Joe's
- Ironman Triathlon Bar by Twin Laboratories, Inc.
- P. R. Bar by P. R. Nutrition, Inc.
- New Vision 40-30-30 Bar by New Vision International, Inc.

Tip: Beware of many nutrition bars! For many years nutrition bars were far too high in carbohydrates, but now many of the bars are loaded with too much protein. If a nutrition bar is too high in carbohydrates, blood sugar levels spike, increasing insulin. Rather than burning fat, your body is forced to burn glucose and store fat. If a nutrition bar is too low in fat, it will not keep you full. But it can be even worse if a nutrition bar is too high in protein, which can cause ketosis and slow the fat burning process. Excess protein can also convert into fat and will be stored in your fat cells. Many high protein, low carbohydrate bars have been made to taste sweet with artificial sweeteners.

40-30-30 SHAKE MIXES

40-30-30 powdered shake mixes make following the Formula even easier. They can be the ultimate liquid fast food. These convenient meal replacement drinks are just like the nutrition bars but in a powdered form. Simply mix the appropriate amount of powder, water, and ice to make a creamy and delicious 40-30-30 shake. We use 40-30-30 powdered shake mixes for a quick meal or snack when we're running late.

Listed below is an approximate nutritional profile for a 40-30-30 powdered drink mix:

40-30-30 POWDERED DRINK MIX

NUTRITIONAL PROFILE (PER SERVING)

Calories:	180–200
Carbohydrates:	20 grams
Protein:	14 grams
Fat:	6 grams

Several companies make 40-30-30 powdered drink mixes. Look for the Balance Bar Company and PR* Nutrition brands. They offer a variety of flavors that taste great.

Tip: Beware of many powdered drink mixes! Many powdered drink mixes are too high in carbohydrates or are loaded with protein. If a powdered drink mix is too high in carbohydrates, blood sugar levels spike, increasing insulin. Rather than burning fat, your body is forced to burn glucose and store fat. If a powdered drink mix is too low in fat, it will not keep you full. But it can be even worse when powdered drink mixes are primarily protein, which can cause ketosis and slow the fat burning process. Excess protein can also convert into fat and will be stored in your fat cells. Many high protein, low carbohydrate drink mixes use low quality protein sources and have been made to taste sweet with artificial sweeteners.

PURE WHEY PROTEIN POWDER

Pure whey protein powder is one of nature's very best proteins. It is a high quality protein that is very easy to digest. Pure whey protein is the newest generation of protein powder and contains an impressive amino acid profile for building and repairing your body when compared to other proteins. Pure whey protein powder mixes instantly and has no chalky aftertaste like many other protein powders. It is basically tasteless and works extremely well when used in specific recipes and desserts.

Tip: Use the 90% rule! When shopping for a pure whey protein powder, look for one that contains pure protein and nothing else. Many protein powders contain carbohydrates and fat as well as artificial sweeteners and flavors.

To determine the percentage of purity of a protein powder, take the total serving size in grams and multiply by .90. The total is what the total grams of protein should be. There should only be one gram or less of carbohydrate and fat. The very best whey protein powders are 90% pure protein.

Listed below is the nutritional profile of the 90% pure whey protein powder that we use in all of our recipes. Use this sample profile when shopping for whey protein powder.

PURE WHEY PROTEIN POWDER

Serving size: 1 scoop (22.2 grams)

Calories: 80

Carbohydrates: 0 grams

Protein: 20 grams

Fat: 0 grams

¼ scoop = 5 grams, ⅓ scoop = 7 grams, ½ scoop = 10 grams, ⅔ scoop = 13 grams, ¾ scoop = 15 grams, 1 scoop = 20 grams

If you have trouble finding a pure whey protein powder, call Craig Nutraceuticals, Inc., at 800-293-1683. Ask for Pure WPI by Bioplex Nutrition, the whey protein powder that the Daousts use in their recipes.

We make a big deal out of emphasizing pure whey protein because when you start shopping for protein powder you will be amazed at all of the hype and different kinds that are now available. There are proteins from milk, whey, casein, soy, egg, egg whites, and more. To help you cut through all of the confusion, just remember the 90% rule. You want a pure protein powder that is 90% protein.

VITAMINS AND MINERALS

Because vitamins and minerals have been depleted in much of the food available today, it's a good idea to use a vitamin and mineral supplement. The quality of supplements can vary, and there are many to choose from, but we are often asked to recommend products by name. Although there are many quality manufacturers, we personally use Montiff products. They are the highest quality available and supply unique balanced formulas of vitamins, minerals, antioxidants, and amino acids. Montiff products have been designed by Don Tyson, one of the world's experts in amino acid formulas and nutraceuticals. We believe Montiff products are the highest quality supplements available.

You can find 40-30-30 Nutrition Bars and powdered shake mixes in health food stores and many grocery stores. Pure WPI whey protein powder and Montiff supplements can be ordered from Craig Nutraceuticals, Inc. They supply many different brands and can be contacted at the number listed below.

Craig Nutraceuticals, Inc.
Nutritional Supplement Hot Line
1-800-293-1683

ABOUT THE AUTHORS

GENE and JOYCE DAOUST are two of the original nutritionists who helped develop and test the 40-30-30 zone nutrition program. In 1992, the Daousts opened the BioSyn Human Performance Center, a cutting-edge weight-loss and sports-nutrition facility and the world's first 40-30-30 zone nutrition clinic. The Daousts frequently appear as featured speakers and conduct programs for corporations nationwide.